✓ GALLUP

MAJOR TRENDS & EVENTS

The Pulse of Our Nation: 1900 to the Present

Obesity

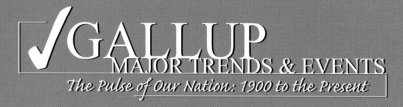

GALLUP
MAJOR TRENDS & EVENTS
The Pulse of Our Nation: 1900 to the Present

Abortion

Drug & Alcohol Abuse

Health Care

Immigration

Marriage & Family Issues

Obesity

Race Relations

Technology

GALLUP
MAJOR TRENDS & EVENTS
The Pulse of Our Nation: 1900 to the Present

Obesity

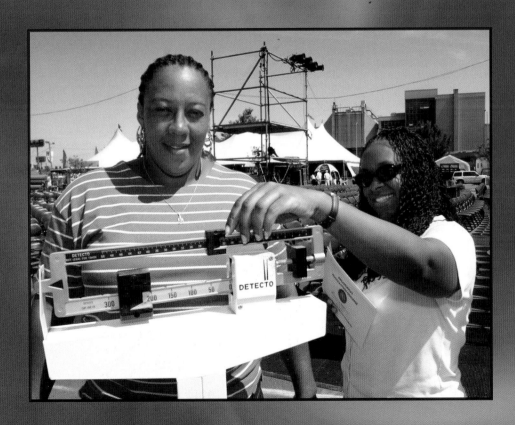

Meg Greene

Produced by OTTN Publishing, Stockton, New Jersey

Mason Crest Publishers
370 Reed Road
Broomall, PA 19008
www.masoncrest.com

3 5 7 9 8 6 4 2

Library of Congress Cataloging-in-Publication Data

Greene, Meg.
    Obesity / Meg Greene.
      p. cm. —— (Gallup major trends and events)
    Includes bibliographical references and index.
    ISBN-13: 978-1-59084-967-5 (hard cover)
    ISBN-10: 1-59084-967-1 (hard cover)
    1. Obesity—Juvenile literature.   I. Title. II. Series.
RA645.O23G74 2006
616.3'98—dc22
                                        2005016313

TABLE OF CONTENTS

Introduction

By Alec Gallup, Chairman, The Gallup Poll

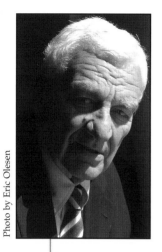

Photo by Eric Olesen

In ways both obvious and subtle, the United States of today differs significantly from the United States that existed at the turn of the 20th century. In 1900, for example, America had not yet taken its place among the world's most influential nations; today the United States stands by itself as the globe's lone superpower. The 1900 census counted about 76 million Americans, largely drawn from white European peoples such as the English, Irish, and Germans; 100 years later the U.S. population was approaching 300 million, and one in every eight residents was of Hispanic origin. In the first years of the 20th century, American society offered women few opportunities to pursue professional careers, and, in fact, women had not yet gained the right to vote. Though slavery had been abolished, black Americans 100 years ago continued to be treated as second-class citizens, particularly in the South, where the Jim Crow laws that would endure for another half-century kept the races separate and unequal.

The physical texture and the pace of American life, too, were much different 100 years ago—or, for that matter, even 50 years ago. Accelerating technological and scientific progress, a hallmark of modern times, has made possible a host of innovations that Americans today take for granted but that would have been unimaginable three generations ago—from brain scans to microwave ovens to cell phones, laptop computers, and the Internet.

No less important than the material, social, and political changes the United States has witnessed over the past century are the changes in American attitudes and perceptions. For example, the way Americans relate to their government and their fellow citizens, how they view marriage and child-rearing norms, where they set the boundary between society's responsibilities and the individual's rights and freedoms—all are key components of Americans' evolving understanding of their nation and its place in the world.

The books in this series examine important issues that have perennially concerned (and sometimes confounded) Americans since the turn of the 20th century. Each volume draws on an array of sources to provide vivid detail and historical context. But, as suggested by the series title, GALLUP MAJOR TRENDS AND EVENTS: THE PULSE OF OUR NATION, 1900 TO THE PRESENT, these books make particular use of the Gallup Organization's vast archive of polling data.

There is perhaps no better source for tracking and understanding American public opinion than Gallup, a name that has been synonymous with opinion polling for seven decades. Over the years, Gallup has elicited responses from more than 3.5 million people on more than 125,000 questions. In 1936 the organization, then known as the American Institute of Public Opinion, emerged into the spotlight when it correctly predicted that Franklin Roosevelt would be reelected president of the United States. This directly contradicted the well-respected Literary Digest Poll, which had announced that Alfred Landon, governor of Kansas, would not only become president but would win in a landslide. Since then Gallup polls have not simply been a fixture in election polling and analysis; they have also cast light on public opinion regarding a broad variety of social, economic, and cultural issues.

Polling results tend to be most noticed during political campaigns or in the wake of important events; during these times, polling provides snapshots of public opinion. This series, however, is more concerned with long-term attitude trends than with responses to breaking news. Thus data from many years of Gallup polls are used to trace the evolution of American attitudes. How, for example, have Americans historically viewed immigration? Did attitudes toward foreign newcomers shift during the Great Depression, after the 1941 Japanese attack on Pearl Harbor, or after the terrorist attacks of September 11, 2001? Do opinions on immigration vary across different age, gender, and ethnic groups?

Or, taking another particularly divisive issue treated in this series, what did Americans think about abortion during the many decades the procedure was generally illegal? How has public opinion changed since the Supreme Court's landmark 1973 *Roe v. Wade* decision? How many Americans now favor overturning *Roe*?

By understanding where we as a society have been, we can better understand where we are—and, sometimes, where we are going.

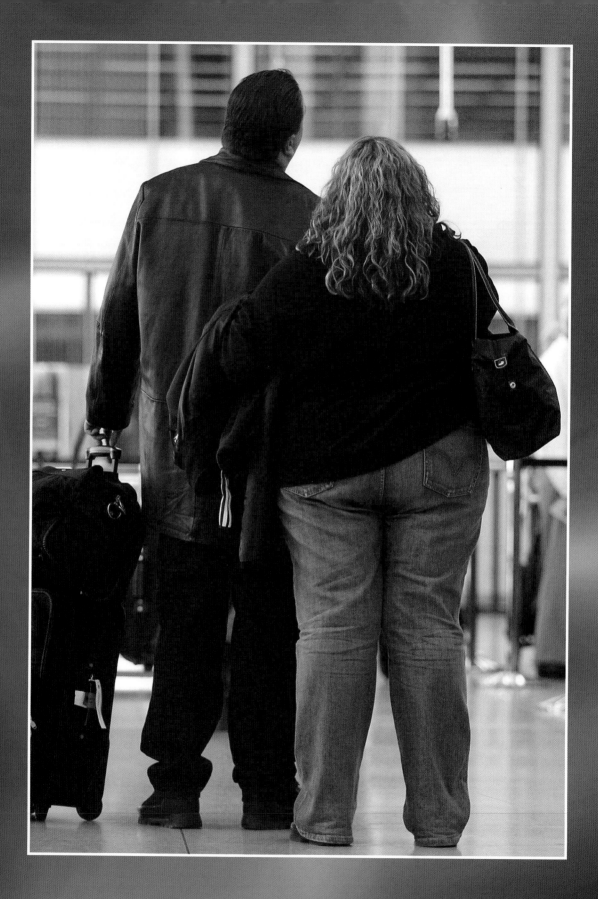

1

THE SWELLING OF AMERICA

During the fall of 1996, an English journalist named Paul Barker visited the United States. While in Washington, D.C., Barker spent an afternoon walking around the National Mall. He was struck by how fat Americans had become since his last visit three years earlier. "I have never seen so many obese people in one place," he wrote in *New Statesman*. "Not plump: obese. In the hot sun everyone wears the uniform of T-shirts, long shorts and trainers. The result is a gross parody of the obsession with health. . . . Bellies overhang. Thighs can barely squeeze past each other. Faces peep out comically from among the jowls and multiple chins of both men and women, and (from about the age of ten) of children also. On a rough reckoning 20 per cent of the (mostly white) people roaming the Mall are like this. I was last in America in 1993. The numbers, or rather the people, have visibly swelled in three years."

Barker's observations were on target. What another writer, Cathy Newman, called "the broadening of America" has become too evident to deny, as more Americans are now dangerously

(Opposite) Americans are heavier today than ever before. The increase in average weight (25 pounds since 1960) has been substantial enough, a recent government study suggests, to translate into higher fuel consumption by airlines.

9

overweight. On average, American men and women are now 25 pounds heavier than were their counterparts in 1960, according to statistics compiled by the Centers for Disease Control and Prevention (CDC) in 2002. The average weight for an American man between the ages of 20 and 74 stood at 166.3 pounds in 1960; by 2002 the figure had risen to 191 pounds. During the same period, the average weight of American women in the 20–74 age group went from 140 pounds to 164.3 pounds. Twenty years ago, a person who weighed 300 pounds was a rarity. Today, doctors report that such patients are common. And the trend in weight gain is continuing, with more Americans overweight today than at any time in the past.

What are the consequences of being overweight or obese? Study after study shows that excess weight takes a terrible toll on the human body. The more weight a person gains, the greater the risk of heart disease, high blood pressure, stroke, diabetes, infertility, gallbladder disease, and osteoarthritis, to say nothing of some forms of cancer. In an article published in 2004 in *JAMA – The Journal of the American Medical Association*, authors Ali H. Mokdad, PhD; James S. Marks, MD, MPH; Donna F. Stroup, PhD, MSc; and Julie L. Gerberding, MD, MPH reported the results of their study of the actual causes of death in the United States in the year 2000. Using mortality data from the CDC, the researchers concluded that an estimated 400,000 deaths were attributable to overweight/obesity (combined with physical inactivity), making it the second-leading cause of preventable deaths in the United States (behind only tobacco use, responsible for an estimated 435,000 deaths in 2000). In addition, the authors suggested that obesity might soon overtake smoking as the number-one cause of preventable death. (It should be noted, however, that other scientists have disputed these conclusions.)

Aside from causing dire health consequences and even death, excess weight and obesity have sizable financial ramifications as well: by 2004, the total annual medical costs for weight-related illnesses in the United States came to an estimated $117 billion—more than the gross domestic product of Costa Rica and Bulgaria combined.

THE BODY MASS INDEX

The word *obese* has become familiar. Yet, many Americans remain uncertain about how being obese is different from merely being overweight. The distinction is important, for it can mean the difference between life and death. As defined by doctors and nutritionists, *obesity* refers to excess body weight in the form of fat. Thus, people are obese when their body fat exceeds a fixed percentage, adjusted for age and sex, of their body weight. For instance, a 25-year-old woman is obese when her body fat is more than 25 percent of her total weight; a 50-year-old woman is obese when her body fat exceeds 30 percent of her total weight. By contrast, a 25-year-old man is considered obese when his body fat makes up more than 20 percent of his total weight; for a 50-year-old man, the threshold is 30 percent of body weight.

Insurance tables, which accounted for height as well as body type (large, medium, or small frame), were among the first tools used to calculate an individual's ideal weight. Today, health-care providers use a slightly more complex formula known as the body mass index (BMI) to determine whether a person is normal, overweight, or obese. The BMI applies a mathematical formula based on a person's height and weight, dividing the person's weight in kilograms by height in meters squared: $BMI = kg/m^2$.

A normal BMI falls between 19 and 24.9. A BMI of 25 to 29.9 indicates that a person is overweight. A person having a BMI of 30 or higher is obese. Those persons who are approximately 100 pounds overweight, or have a BMI of 40 or above, are deemed "morbidly obese." Although the BMI is not perfect (it does not, for instance, take into account the difference between fat and muscle in determining body mass), it does offer an approximate guide to determine obesity, which enables doctors to predict the development of health problems related to weight.

Body Mass Index (BMI) Table

BMI	19	20	21	22	23	24	25	26	27	28	29	30	31	32	33	34	35
Height								*Weight (in pounds)*									
4'10" (58")	91	96	100	105	110	115	119	124	129	134	138	143	148	153	158	162	167
4'11" (59")	94	99	104	109	114	119	124	128	133	138	143	148	153	158	163	168	173
5' (60")	97	102	107	112	118	123	128	133	138	143	148	153	158	163	168	174	179
5'1" (61")	100	106	111	116	122	127	132	137	143	148	153	158	164	169	174	180	185
5'2" (62")	104	109	115	120	126	131	136	142	147	153	158	164	169	175	180	186	191
5'3" (63")	107	113	118	124	130	135	141	146	152	158	163	169	175	180	186	191	197
5'4" (64")	110	116	122	128	134	140	145	151	157	163	169	174	180	186	192	197	204
5'5" (65")	114	120	126	132	138	144	150	156	162	168	174	180	186	192	198	204	210
5'6" (66")	118	124	130	136	142	148	155	161	167	173	179	186	192	198	204	210	216
5'7" (67")	121	127	134	140	146	153	159	166	172	178	185	191	198	204	211	217	223
5'8" (68")	125	131	138	144	151	158	164	171	177	184	190	197	203	210	216	223	230
5'9" (69")	128	135	142	149	155	162	169	176	182	189	196	203	209	216	223	230	236
5'10" (70")	132	139	146	153	160	167	174	181	188	195	202	209	216	222	229	236	243
5'11" (71")	136	143	150	157	165	172	179	186	193	200	208	215	222	229	236	243	250
6' (72")	140	147	154	162	169	177	184	191	199	206	213	221	228	235	242	250	258
6'1" (73")	144	151	159	166	174	182	189	197	204	212	219	227	235	242	250	257	265
6'2' (74")	148	155	163	171	179	186	194	202	210	218	225	233	241	249	256	264	272
6'3' (75")	152	160	168	176	184	192	200	208	216	224	232	240	248	256	264	272	279

Source: Evidence Report of Clinical Guidelines on the Identification, Evaluation, and Treatment of Overweight and Obesity in Adults, 1998. NIH/National Heart, Lung, and Blood Institute (NHLBI)

The body mass index (BMI) is a tool for measuring whether a person falls into the normal weight, over-weight, or obese category. An adult with a BMI of 25 or above is considered overweight, while an adult with a BMI of 30 or above is classified as obese. It should be remembered, however, that these categories can be somewhat imprecise because BMI doesn't distinguish between muscle and fat in overall weight.

S. O. S., OR SOBERING OBESITY STATISTICS

In a Gallup poll conducted in November 2005, about 4 in 10 American adults described themselves as overweight (with nearly 37 percent saying they were "somewhat" overweight, and 5 percent saying they were "very" overweight). The actual numbers may be considerably higher, however: the National Center for Health Statistics (NCHS), using data from the period 1999–2002, estimates that 64 percent of Americans age 20 and older are overweight, with 30 percent falling into the obese category.

Nor is the problem confined to adults. According to the CDC, an estimated 9 million American children and teens age 6 to 19 — about 16 percent of the individuals in that age group — are overweight. And that percentage has more than tripled, the CDC says, since 1980. Excess weight is even a concern among the preschool set: some 10 percent of children ages two to five are classified as overweight. Some doctors predict that individuals in this generation may be the first to die before their parents. As one pediatrician said in 2004: "We're leading a race we shouldn't want to win."

Obesity is a problem that cuts across gender, race, and class lines. But more women (33 percent) than men (28 percent) are obese, and among women obesity is more prevalent in blacks (49 percent) and Hispanics (38 percent) than in whites (31 percent). Obesity used to be seen as a problem predominantly affecting the lower classes. While the unemployed and the working poor are still the most likely to suffer from obesity, the problem has become much more prevalent among middle-class and wealthy Americans. Over the past few decades, in fact, rates of obesity have shown a particularly dramatic rise among college-educated Americans ages 18 to 29 years.

The obesity problem also is compounded by the fact that members of the baby-boomer generation (those born between 1945 and 1965) often deny that added weight constitutes a severe health problem for themselves, their children, or their grandchildren. In his book *Fat Land: How Americans Became the Fattest People in the World*, Greg Critser observes: "Get a group of Baby Boomers together and, within minutes, the topic of obesity shifts not to medical issues, but, rather, to aesthetic and gender issues, to the notion—widely held in the urban upper middle class—that 'talking too much about obesity just ends up making kids have low self-esteem.' "

THE SILENT EPIDEMIC

The CDC has labeled obesity in the United States an epidemic. But until recently, policymakers and the public paid scant attention to the warnings sounded by doctors and researchers. The noted psychologist Kelly D. Brownell, author of the 2004 book *Food Fight: The Inside Story of the Food Industry, America's Obesity Crisis and What We Can Do About It*, observes that the obesity epidemic "came quickly, with little fanfare, and was out of control before the nation noticed." As early as 1961, health officials warned that the number of obese Americans was growing, elevating the risk of diabetes, heart disease, and related ailments. By 1962 the U.S. Department of Agriculture estimated that, on average, Americans ate almost 1,488 pounds of food per year, with the most gluttonous eating approximately 8 pounds of food a day. That same year, the number of obese Americans was estimated at 48 million.

By 1980, an estimated 46 percent of American adults were overweight. In the 25 years that followed, the average weight of American adults increased by nearly 1 percent per year. The result? Today the proportion of overweight Americans approaches two-thirds.

Alarmed by the recent trends and statistics, many Americans have begun to search for answers. Meanwhile health officials, doctors, psychologists, and

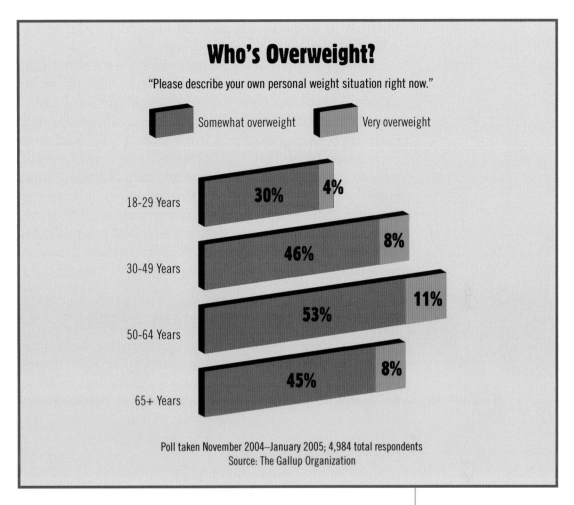

Who's Overweight?

"Please describe your own personal weight situation right now."

■ Somewhat overweight   ■ Very overweight

18-29 Years   30%   4%

30-49 Years   46%   8%

50-64 Years   53%   11%

65+ Years   45%   8%

Poll taken November 2004–January 2005; 4,984 total respondents
Source: The Gallup Organization

nutritionists have increased efforts to educate a nation once blissfully unaware of, and perhaps indifferent to, a threat that, some believe, could become one of the gravest medical crises this country has ever faced.

Aside from health and financial ramifications, obesity and being overweight have other consequences. People who are overweight are seen and, in many cases, treated differently. Obesity carries a stigma, even though more Americans are now overweight. A recent study at Michigan State University asked undergraduates whether they would be more inclined to marry an embezzler, a cocaine addict, or an obese person. A vast majority of respondents preferred the embezzler or the addict to someone who was obese.

Whatever people's perceptions on excess weight, many businesses and industries have had to make adjustments to account for Americans' growing girth. For instance, the ferries that operate in Puget Sound, carrying passengers to and from Seattle, have widened their seats from 18 to 20 inches to allow overweight people some measure of comfort. In Colorado, some ambulances are now equipped with a winch (a machine for lifting loads) and a plus-size compartment to serve patients weighing up to half a ton (1,000 pounds). An Indiana casket manufacturer offers an oversized model, measuring 38 inches wide, compared with the standard 24 inches.

THE PUBLIC AND POLITICIANS RESPOND

The good news is that more Americans are becoming aware of the health problems associated with being overweight and obese. In a survey conducted in 2004, for example, Americans rated obesity, alongside heart disease, cancer, AIDS, and drug abuse, as among the nation's most pressing public health concerns. In a Gallup poll conducted that same year, more than 61 percent of the respondents said they wanted to lose weight. Yet only about 28 percent said they were currently taking serious steps to do so.

For the majority of Americans, the solution to combating obesity is uncomplicated: eat less and exercise more. But the solution, while simple to identify, is not easy to implement in a nation inundated by prepared foods and prone to sedentary work habits and limited physical activity. In an effort to surmount such obstacles, Americans spend billions of dollars every year on weight-loss products, nutritional programs, exercise equipment, and health-club memberships. Those who are morbidly obese may take more drastic measures, including liposuction (surgery that removes fat deposits in a localized area) or gastric bypass surgery (which reduces the body's caloric intake), of which more than 100,000 procedures were performed between 2003 and 2004. Food and drug companies also spend millions of dollars in research to develop drugs that will melt the pounds away. Yet, despite these efforts, "the nation's collective waistline," as writer Michael Lemonick put it in a 2004 *Time* magazine article, "just keeps growing."

By 2000 obesity had expanded from being a health problem to a political issue. In May 2002 a $4.1 million USDA Team Nutrition program began teaching children healthy eating habits, while the White House Health and Fitness Initiative emphasized physical activity. Medicare redefined obesity as a medical problem, opening the door for Medicare recipients to be covered for obesity surgery and hospital programs that provide diet and exercise management. The Social Security Administration proposed allowing obese individuals to qualify for disability income. Even the Internal Revenue Service got involved, recognizing the importance of treating obesity by allowing taxpayers enrolled in physician-prescribed weight-loss programs to deduct their medical expenses beginning in April 2002.

The problem of obesity also found a place in the domestic agenda of President George W. Bush. On March 12, 2004, President Bush announced a campaign to combat the obesity epidemic. Later that day, Tommy Thompson, secretary of the Department of Health and Human Services, held a news conference in which he encouraged Americans to undertake "small steps" to better health by eating less and exercising more. Thompson also called for voluntary measures—for restaurants to put calorie information on menus and for food companies to provide accurate calorie counts on product labels. These steps, Thompson noted, marked the beginning of the government's "commitment to

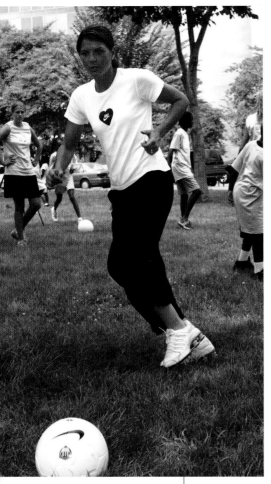

A variety of public and private initiatives have recently targeted the rising rates of childhood obesity in the United States. In this July 2003 photo, soccer legend Mia Hamm helps kick off the "Get Kids in Action" program, sponsored by the University of North Carolina and Gatorade.

reversing this tragic obesity trend in which far too many Americans are literally eating themselves to death."

TRUE CRISIS?

Still, not all Americans are convinced that the public is in danger because of obesity. A recent bombshell involving the obesity epidemic exploded in April 2005, when the respected *Journal of the American Medical Association* published its own estimates of how many deaths can be attributed to obesity and related illnesses per year. *JAMA* estimated the annual number of obesity-related deaths in the United States at just 25,814—some 14 times lower than the then-current CDC estimate. If accurate, the *JAMA* figure would rank obesity seventh, not second, among the leading causes of death, behind car crashes and gunshot wounds. While the CDC, later in 2005, revised downward its estimate of annual deaths associated with obesity, its figure of 112,000 remained far higher than the *JAMA* estimate.

The huge disparities reflect the difficulty of assessing the consequences of a condition that does not by itself produce death but that contributes to numerous other conditions that may. "Because obesity has so many different effects on so many diseases," the CDC explained, "it is extremely difficult for doctors to identify obesity-related deaths reliably on death certificates. So, instead, scientists use complex modeling techniques to estimate deaths related to obesity."

As a result of the great disparity in the figures, however, a lively and sometimes hostile debate has evolved over whether or not an obesity crisis even exists.

Regardless of whether there is a crisis or a smaller problem, blame is cast at various sources, from the fast-food companies to the grocery industry to the health profession to individuals shirking personal responsibility. Not even the government is immune from all the finger-pointing. As the debate rages on, one thing is certain: some Americans are eating way too much, exercising way too little, and paying a high price for both.

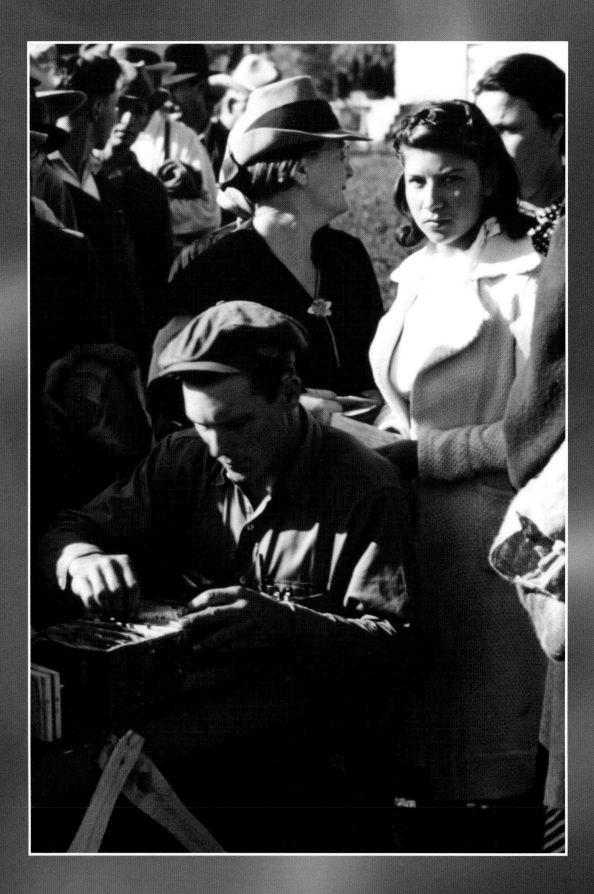

2

A NATION'S GROWING APPETITE

How did a people who only five decades ago were considered among the healthiest in the world become the fattest? The obvious answer is that many Americans acquired the habit of eating too much and not exercising enough. The solution seems equally obvious: change eating and exercise habits. Yet, despite warnings and incentives, many Americans thus far have not improved their behaviors. Instead, government and health officials, as well as average citizens, have sought scapegoats, whether the fast-food restaurants or the manufacturers of processed food.

History may provide some insight into the problem. Until the last 200 years or so, most of the people in the world endured regular food shortages. (The last great famine in Europe in which people starved to death occurred during the 1840s, and in much of Africa and other parts of the so-called Third World today malnutrition and starvation are chronic.) When presented with the opportunity to eat to their fill, therefore, people usually did so with gusto. Since human physiology has remained almost

(Opposite) Residents of St. Johns, Arizona, wait in line for food handouts toward the end of the Great Depression. Today prosperity, more sedentary lifestyles, an abundance of leisure time, and the easy availability of processed (and often high-fat) foods have combined to make Americans the world's fattest people.

unchanged for thousands of years, people still love to eat. But circumstances are different. An act that was once a matter of survival has, ironically, become detrimental to health in a world where many now have plenty.

THE APPETITE FOR SURVIVAL

In the past, most people struggled to find enough to eat. As a consequence of this and other hardships, life expectancy was short. In Europe until at least the mid-17th century, for example, men reaching 40 and women reaching 30 were an anomaly. They were uncommonly old and probably looked it. The best-fed members of medieval society — kings, princes, and patricians — died on average between 45 and 56 years of age. Fifty-two years old in 1514, King Louis XII of France was considered "*fort débile et antique*," very old and decrepit. Of all the dangers that men and women faced in this earlier age, obesity and its related illnesses were nowhere to be found.

The diet of ordinary people, which included the majority of the population, consisted of fruit (mainly pears and apples), roots, wild nuts, garlic, onions, and other vegetables, though the last were rarely eaten fresh but reserved for use in soups and stews. The staple food was pulse (which is similar to a lentil bean) and rough, black bread. Only the wealthy could afford rye or wheat flour. Until the end of the 18th century, most people in Europe used wild honey rather than sugar as a sweetener. A diet deficient not only in calories, but also in essential fats, vitamins, minerals, and proteins led to widespread malnutrition and disease.

Our primate ancestors were not meat eaters. Some 2.5 million years ago, however, the genus *Homo* (which includes modern humans) emerged. Brain size increased substantially, and the human brain grew more complex. Many anthropologists now believe that this relatively rapid growth of the human brain, which was crucial to the overall evolution of human beings into a more sophisticated species, is associated with the addition of meat to the diet. Meat, unlike the nuts, roots, and tubers that other primates subsisted on, was rich in calories and protein to fuel the developing human brain.

Additionally, both sweets and fats were added to the human diet; their tastes were attractive, and for good reason. As Daniel Benyshek, a professor of anthropology, points out: "It makes sense [that] evolution would select for those desires. We acquired a taste for fatty foods because they have more calories per gram, and (sweetness) is a good general signal nature gives that a product is a high-calorie food."

EARLY EATING PATTERNS

A recent study estimates that to survive, early ancestors of modern man (*Homo sapiens*), known variously as *Homo erectus*, *Homo habilis*, and *Homo ergaster*, had to consume between 4,000 and 10,000 calories daily, far more than we need today. Our early ancestors did not grow obese, however, since the calories they consumed were rapidly spent. These people did not live sedentary lives.

The search for food itself was difficult and grueling, requiring great physical strength and endurance. Hunting, which was indispensable to supplementing the diet, required that the prey be tracked, sometimes over long distances, caught, and killed. Also, the quest for fruits, nuts, roots, and vegetables was not a pleasant outing but a difficult undertaking that often required climbing or digging. Then, too, world temperatures during the emergence of modern humans (between 150,000 and 100,000 years ago) were often markedly lower than they are today, and simply keeping warm could require expending an enormous amount of energy.

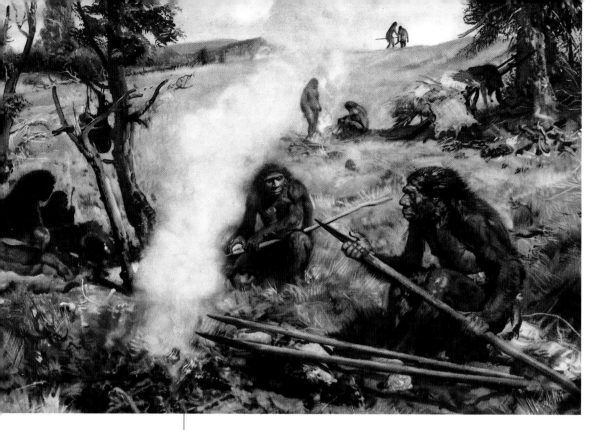

Neanderthals fabricate
weapons for hunting.
Some scientists believe
that our taste for high-fat
foods is the result of hundreds of thousands of
years of evolution: in the
grueling world of our
hominid ancestors, fats
would have been the rich-
est source of the calories
necessary for survival.

THE AGRICULTURAL REVOLUTION

One of the most important technological breakthroughs in history was the development of agriculture. As human beings became more settled and sophisticated, they gradually learned how to grow some of their own food. In time, farmers produced enough food to feed themselves and their families and then to sustain small agricultural communities. Especially fertile harvests might even produce a surplus beyond immediate needs.

While the development of agriculture made possible human civilization, the switch to a more settled lifestyle did not come without certain negative health consequences. As journalist Michael D. Lemonick pointed out in his *Time* article, some anthropologists argue that although agriculture provided people with access to a steady food supply, at the same time, diets became less nutritious. The growing reliance on grains, such as wheat and oats, actually made for a less healthy population, these scientists believe. Evidence for this assertion can be found in the skeletons of early farmers, which show a greater presence of calcium deficiency, anemia, and bacterial infections, for example. (Of course, it must be noted that average life spans also increased as a result of the more reliable food supply.)

Eventually, domesticated animals replaced wild game as the chief source of meat. This caused fat intake to increase, as wild game contains much less fat. Herds of cattle and goats also provided fatty dairy products, which over time contributed to heart disease and other circulatory ailments. Still, despite these changes, obesity was rarely a problem as people remained active in daily life, a pattern that continued until the last decades of the 19th century, when in the advanced countries "brain work" began to replace manual labor.

THE AMERICAN WAY OF EATING

Another way to understand how obesity emerged as one of the leading health concerns of the 21st century is to look specifically to the American past. Until the late 19th century, Americans' way of eating consisted of distinct regional traditions brought mostly from England, Scotland, Ireland, and Africa, and to a lesser extent from Holland, Germany, and Scandinavia (few persons of European ancestry adopted the diets of Native Americans). Immigrants tended to cling to their culinary traditions as a way to maintain ties to the old country. But as English colonists began intermingling with immigrant peoples of other cultures and races, they were introduced to a variety of new ingredients and different foods. This contact brought about dishes that combined old and new.

Before the Civil War (1861–1865), there were four major food traditions in the United States, each with English roots. These included a New England tradition that associated plain cooking with religious piety. Hostile toward fancy or highly seasoned foods, which they regarded as a sinful form of sensual indulgence, New Englanders adopted an austere diet stressing boiled and baked meats, boiled vegetables, and baked breads and pies. A Southern tradition, with its more elaborate seasonings and its emphasis on frying and simmering, was an amalgam of African, English, French, Spanish, and Indian culinary techniques. In the middle-Atlantic region, influenced by Quakerism, the diet again tended to be plain and simple. In the backcountry, the diet included many ingredients that the English commonly used as animal feed, such as potatoes, corn, and various greens. The frontier diet also stressed griddle cakes, grits, fish, game, pork, and dried beef.

One distinctive aspect of the traditional American diet was the abundance of meat. As Americans moved westward, open plains and grasslands encouraged the feeding of large herds of cattle, pigs, and sheep. With the arrival of large groups of German immigrants in the 19th century, Americans were introduced to a wide array of marinated meats, sausages, and meat pastries, as well as such popular foods as barbecued chicken, beef, and pork; hot dogs; and hamburgers.

By the late 19th century, more food was being processed and mass-produced. Whereas American housewives once had done all the food preparation for their families, now a growing variety of precooked, preserved, canned, and packaged foods appeared on the market. Long before the rise of fast-food chains, processed foods found a place on kitchen tables across the United States. Although many historians attribute the popularity of convenience foods to the feminist movement of the 1960s and 1970s — when more women entered the workplace and, as a result, had less time to prepare meals — the truth is that such processed foods had long been a part of the American diet.

Among the first and most successful food industries were the factories that made processed grains and corn into cereal, such as Kellogg's cereal company of Battle

Creek, Michigan. Established in 1906 by William and John Kellogg, the factory soon began producing hot and cold cereals such as oatmeal and cornflakes. According to John Kellogg, good nutrition was invaluable to health, and he believed that more Americans would enjoy a healthy diet if food preparation were easier. "It often occurred to me," he wrote, "that it should be possible to purchase cereals at groceries already cooked and ready to eat, and I considered different ways in which this might be done." Promoted as one of America's first health foods, cereals quickly became a part of the American breakfast.

By the 1920s other techniques, such as freezing and canning, became more common. These innovations influenced the development of cafeterias and lunch counters, like those established in Woolworth's department stores. Other changes in eating habits occurred in the 1950s, when the interstate highway system was

Workers at a bean cannery, 1934. Preserved and processed foods made life more convenient—but often at the cost of good nutrition.

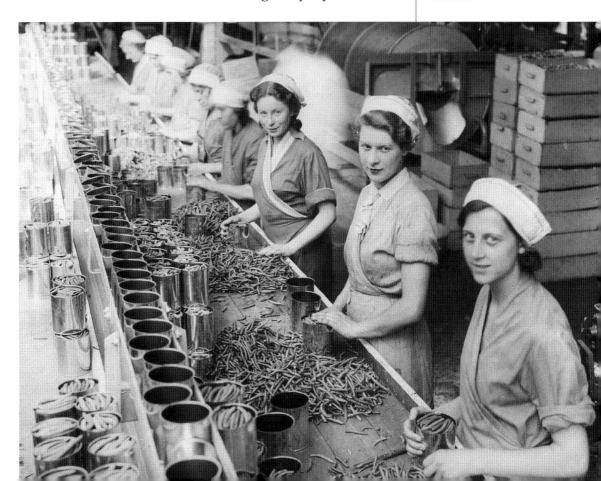

developed and Americans who were on the go began looking for places to grab a quick, inexpensive meal. The result, as one professor has observed, was that America "began to develop a culture of people who liked drive-throughs. We became accustomed to that kind of food," and the fast-food restaurant was born.

CHANGING WORLD, CHANGING APPETITES

Soon fast food became not merely a convenience for travelers but a way of life. Once people had to track, kill, and dress game; slaughter and butcher their own livestock; milk their own cows; churn their own butter; gather their own eggs; harvest their own wheat, barley, rye, or corn; grind their own flour; and bake their own bread. Now they had only to drive to the nearest fast-food restaurant. It was not long before a phone call or e-mail brought prepared food to the front door.

The prevalence of two-income households has also brought about changes in the way Americans eat. Now it is much less common for families to sit down to have home-cooked meals together. According to a December 2003 Gallup poll, only 28 percent of Americans had family dinners seven days a week, compared with 38 percent as recently as 2001. According to the same poll, however, 75 percent of families have dinner together at least four times a week. Yet when these families do dine together, the odds are that they will not be eating a fully home-cooked meal.

Convenience has obviously come at a cost. In addition to being higher in fat and sugar, most prepared and processed foods are loaded with chemicals and preservatives. Still, Americans consume them in abundance. According to a 1965 study, between 27 and 30 percent of American households used convenience foods. By the 1990s convenience foods comprised a large portion of the average diet in the United States. Several studies indicate that many American families now subsist entirely on convenience foods and fast food.

As of 2001 nearly every American household used convenience foods in one form or another. Americans had at their disposal an immense variety of mass-produced, comparatively inexpensive dinners, snacks, candy, and other fat-filled, sugar-laden treats packed with calories but having almost no nutritional value. One health researcher lamented that, as a result, "we've changed the environment that we live in in an incredibly short time—one generation or perhaps two generations at most, and this has challenged our ancient metabolism, which for thousands of generations has been geared to fighting famine."

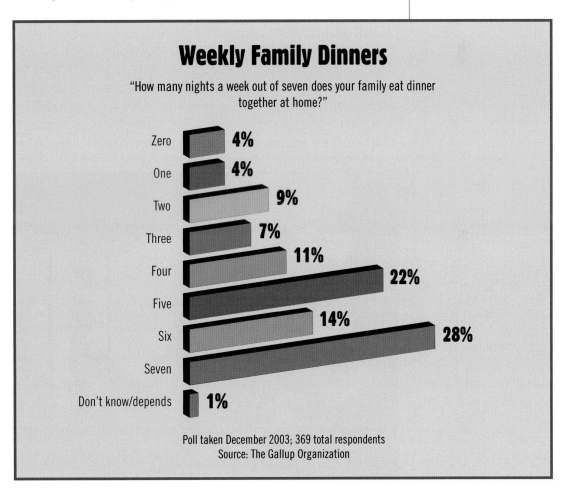

Weekly Family Dinners

"How many nights a week out of seven does your family eat dinner together at home?"

Zero	4%
One	4%
Two	9%
Three	7%
Four	11%
Five	22%
Six	14%
Seven	28%
Don't know/depends	1%

Poll taken December 2003; 369 total respondents
Source: The Gallup Organization

WHAT HAPPENED?

Yet, obesity in America has not been merely the consequence of innovations in food production; there are a number of other factors at work. For instance, the marketing of food in the mass media, particularly television, has saturated children with advertisements touting all manner of fast food, cereal, and candy. Additionally, modern technology—such as the washing machine, the elevator, and even the automatic door—has subtly reduced the calorie-burning activities of Americans in everyday life. Even crime has played a role in the spread of obesity; as violence escalates, people become more afraid to venture outside for a walk or to exercise.

In addition, despite the recent rise in oil and gas prices, many Americans still love their cars. They prefer driving to walking or riding a bicycle. If people live in areas where malls, supermarkets, and shopping centers are not within easy walking distance, or where walking would be dangerous, they also will drive, whatever their preference may be. Finally, many Americans drive

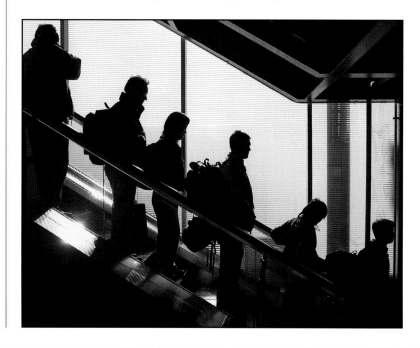

Escalators move travelers at Chicago's O'Hare International Airport. Even subtle changes in the amount of calories people expend in daily life can add up to excess pounds over the long term.

their cars to and from work, which for many is a desk job that requires little physical activity. Of course, Americans also jog, swim, ski, play sports, and go to the gym, but everyday life affords fewer opportunities for exercise than it formerly did.

LINKING PAST AND PRESENT

Changes in the accessibility and technology of food have enabled us to produce more food than we can, and should, eat. Unfortunately, the past has not caught up with the present. A species designed to survive food shortages cannot easily adjust to abundance. As the Rutgers University anthropologist Lionel Tiger has explained, human beings "don't have a cut-off mechanism for eating. Our bodies tell us, 'Fat is good to eat but hard to get.'" Clearly, in advanced countries such as the United States at the beginning of the 21st century, fat is more accessible than ever before, but our bodies and our appetites have not yet become accustomed to the change and adjusted our eating habits accordingly. Daniel Benyshek agrees. In an interview, he stated:

> We really don't have to work at all to access food. What created a balance for our forebears was not only famine, but that they had to work hard to grow, collect, or somehow obtain food. Today, most of us sit at computers all day and drive cars everywhere. We're not burning calories or challenging our aerobic capacity. People don't realize how modest our caloric needs are. They still insist on three good-sized meals a day, plus two or three lattes with sugar, as well as a couple of snacks.

Americans' appetite for food, while rooted in the past, no longer serves its original purpose: survival. With easy access to an apparently unlimited supply of cheap food and machines designed to make the world less physically demanding, Americans have lives that men and women once could only dream about. Ironically, such innovations and advances have produced unforeseen problems, for Americans are now killing themselves with food.

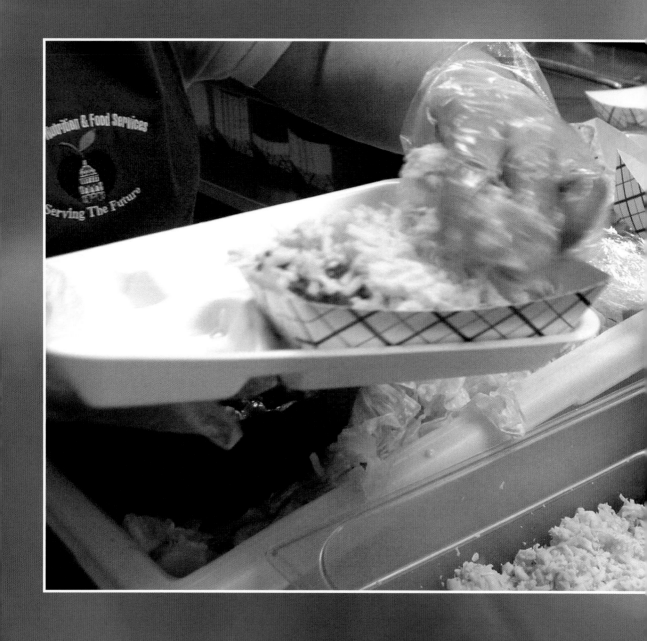

3 THE CAUSES AND COSTS OF OBESITY

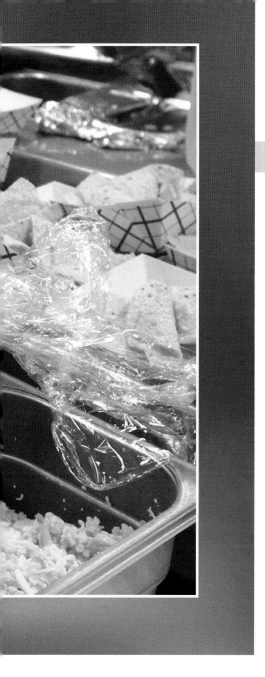

While school districts across the country have tried to offer kids more healthful cafeteria fare, many report that the students continue to prefer high-fat favorites like pizza, fried chicken, and french fries.

n July 2002 newspaper reporter Sally Squires wrote, "Here we are in the 21st century, surrounded by more cheap and plentiful food than has been available since the Garden of Eden, and Americans are still struggling to learn how to eat." Squires emphasized a painful truth. For many researchers and health professionals, understanding the causes of, and cure for, obesity is not easy. Although many people may attribute it to eating too much or to a "fat gene" passed from generation to generation within some families, the reality is far more complicated. Obesity results from a variety of causes; it arises not just from what we eat but also from how, when, and why we eat. To understand and treat the disease, scientists and doctors must therefore consider genetics, diet, and nutrition, as well as psychological and environmental factors.

THE ROLE OF CALORIES IN WEIGHT GAIN

While the causes of obesity may be complex and multifaceted, the actual process of weight gain is fairly straightforward. A person gains weight when his or her body takes in more calories than it uses.

A calorie is a unit of heat that measures the energy content of food. Calories are important; they provide the fuel the body needs to survive and function. When a person is active or ill, the body needs extra calories. However, under ordinary conditions of activity or health, the body stores excess calories as fat, producing weight gain. The amount of weight gain that leads to obesity does not happen in a few weeks or months. Because being obese is more than being only a few pounds overweight, people who suffer from obesity usually have been getting many more calories than they need for years.

The proper caloric intake varies from person to person. People who work at jobs that demand very high levels of physical activity might need as many as 4,000 to 5,000 calories per day to maintain their weight. People whose jobs are more sedentary and who do not exercise may require as few as 1,500 calories per day. Of great concern among health professionals is that Americans today consume more calories than they did 30 years ago and are, in general, less active.

During the 29-year period between 1971 and 2000, according to a 2004 report issued by the National Center for Health Statistics, the average caloric intake of American women increased 22 percent, from 1,542 to 1,877 calories per day. During the same period, the average caloric intake of American men increased 7 percent, from 2,450 to 2,618 calories per day.

Gender seems to play a significant role in weight gain. Men have a leaner body mass than women. As a result, men tend to burn more calories and carry less fat than women. Still, there is no dearth of overweight American men, just as there is no scarcity of overweight American women.

OBESITY'S CAUSES

Obesity tends to run in families. Studies suggest that the children of obese parents are 25 to 30 percent more likely to become obese themselves than are children whose parents are not obese. This leads some people to believe that a "fat gene" must be at work in obesity. Of course, eating and exercise habits also tend to be influenced by one's family, so the matter is not so simple. It is highly likely that, as with other health conditions, obesity is linked to hereditary and environmental factors.

Currently, some studies suggest a genetic link to how a person's body stores and processes fat. If further research firmly establishes that connection, doctors will have an easier time predicting who is at risk for obesity. Again, however, heredity does not explain everything. Researchers also need to consider diet, nutrition, eating habits, level of activity, and even body type.

Body type is known to play a role in obesity. There are three basic human body types: the ectomorph, the endomorph, and the mesomorph. People with an ectomorph shape demonstrate a low capacity for fat storage, so obesity is generally not a concern for them. Endomorphs have the greatest fat-storage capacity, making them more likely candidates to become overweight or obese. A mesomorph's capacity for fat storage falls somewhere in between that of the other two body shapes, but fat is also more evenly distributed on the mesomorph's frame. In reality, most people are a combination of body shapes, with a tendency toward one or another. Hence, experts doubt that body type is the main risk factor for obesity.

One of the more recent medical breakthroughs in fighting obesity has come from studying leptin, a naturally occurring hormone that controls the appetite. Leptin is secreted by fat cells when they are full, which helps to curb appetite. When a body produces too little leptin, fat cells cannot signal the brain that they are full. As a result, people overeat and weight gain occurs. Because leptin inhibits the appetite, it has attracted much attention as a possible treatment for obesity. Preliminary tests have shown that some obese persons lose weight when treated with leptin, but the results are far from conclusive and use of the hormone remains controversial.

In a few cases, obesity is caused by hormonal imbalances or other medical problems. For instance, people with hypothyroidism suffer weight gain because they cannot maintain normal metabolic rates that enable the

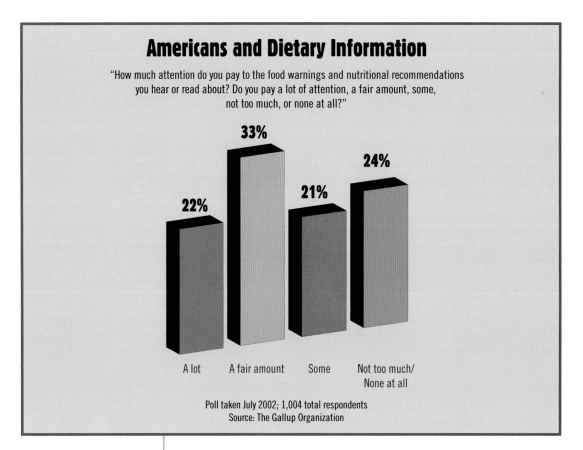

Americans and Dietary Information

"How much attention do you pay to the food warnings and nutritional recommendations you hear or read about? Do you pay a lot of attention, a fair amount, some, not too much, or none at all?"

33%

24%

21%

22%

A lot   A fair amount   Some   Not too much/ None at all

Poll taken July 2002; 1,004 total respondents
Source: The Gallup Organization

body to burn fat. Cushing's syndrome, which causes abnormalities in the production of corticosteroid, also causes weight gain. Depression and certain neurological problems sometimes lead to overeating and weight gain as well. Certain drugs, such as steroids and some antidepressants, also may cause people to put on weight.

By itself, heredity explains the occurrence of obesity in only a small percentage of Americans. Therefore, obesity experts also study how weight is affected by people's environment and behavior, as well as by the general state of their mental and physical health. Clearly, environment is important. One researcher, quoted in Kelly Brownell's book *Food Fight*, commented that "genes load the gun, the environment pulls the trigger." In other words, some people may be predisposed to obesity, but how they live will determine whether they actually become obese. To combat an unhealthy environment that promotes the convenience and taste of prepared and fast foods high in sugar and fat but with little nutritional value, doctors must address bad eating habits as well as heredity.

Recently, doctors and researchers again have begun to consider the connections between physical and mental health. As a result, they have confirmed that various psychological factors influence eating habits and activity levels. Stress, boredom, anger, frustration, and depression may cause some people to overeat, may diminish some people's energy and thus reduce their level of physical activity, and may even slow the body's metabolism, inhibiting its ability to burn fat. Poor

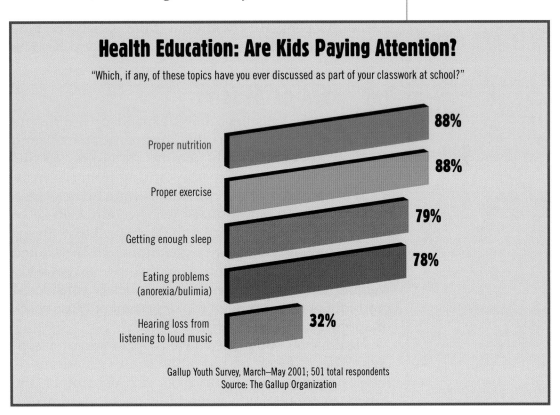

Health Education: Are Kids Paying Attention?

"Which, if any, of these topics have you ever discussed as part of your classwork at school?"

- Proper nutrition — **88%**
- Proper exercise — **88%**
- Getting enough sleep — **79%**
- Eating problems (anorexia/bulimia) — **78%**
- Hearing loss from listening to loud music — **32%**

Gallup Youth Survey, March–May 2001; 501 total respondents
Source: The Gallup Organization

emotional health may thereby contribute to the onset of obesity.

Although research indicates that overweight people have no more psychological problems than people whose height and weight are most closely proportionate, estimates also suggest that 10 percent of those who are obese and try to lose weight have binge eating disorders. During an episode of binging, people eat large quantities of food with no sense of self-control or satisfaction. Those with the most severe binge eating problems are also most likely to have symptoms of depression and low self-esteem. These men and women have difficulty losing weight, and, if they do lose weight, have problems keeping it off. Many trap themselves in a vicious circle. If they fail to lose weight, they can become depressed, which prompts them to binge and gain more weight. As their depression and low self-esteem deepens, they withdraw from society, become more sedentary, binge, gain more weight, and become obese.

THE COSTS OF OBESITY

As American waistlines have expanded, health-care costs have soared, in part due to expenses for treating diseases associated with obesity. According to one study, the health-care expenses arising from the treatment of morbidly obese individuals were twice as high as the costs of treating those who were not obese or overweight. Data compiled in 2000 showed that 10 percent of annual health-care expenditures in the United States, a total of $56 billion, were linked to excess body weight. The nearly 5 million Americans considered morbidly obese accounted for 20 percent of those costs, or approximately $11.2 billion.

Health-care authorities have ample reason for concern. The number of morbidly obese Americans is increasing rapidly: as of 2000, 2.2 percent of the American population was morbidly obese, up from 0.78

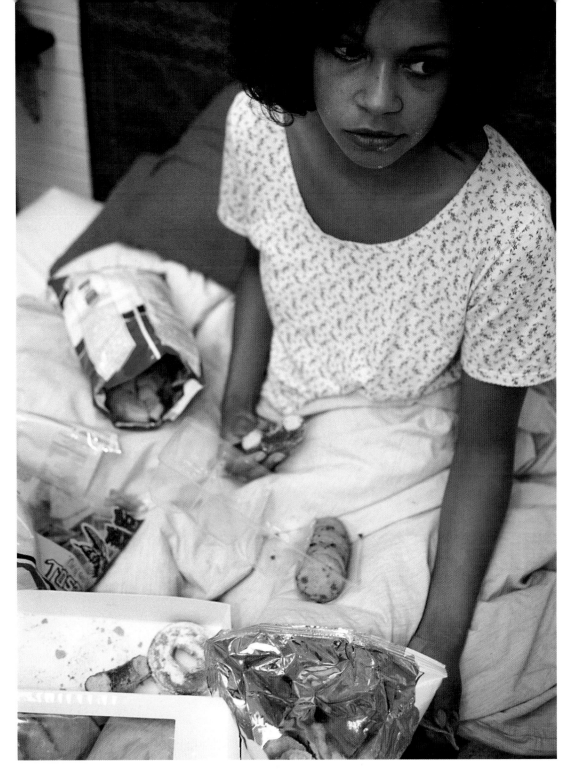

Depression may contribute to various eating problems, such as binge eating.

percent just a decade earlier. By 2004 obesity-related health-care costs amounted to $75 billion, or about 6 percent of all national health expenditures.

Who is paying the bill? According to a 2004 study, nearly half the health-care costs associated with obesity are paid by tax-supported insurance plans such as Medicare or Medicaid. Twenty-one percent of Medicare patients (the vast majority of whom are age 65 or older) are obese. They were responsible for $18 billion in health-care costs, approximately 7 percent of the total

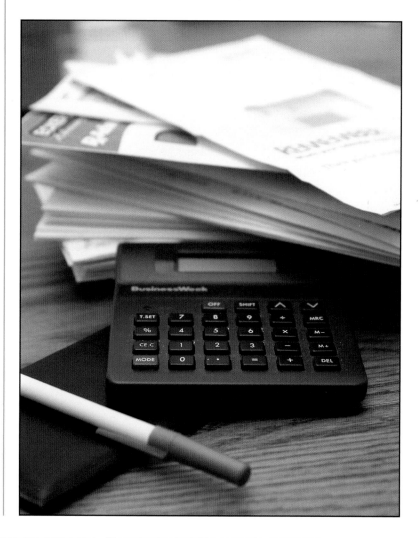

The high cost of treating obesity-related illnesses, some experts believe, threatens to overwhelm the U.S. health-care delivery system.

STAPLING THE STOMACH

For people who are morbidly obese (at least 100 pounds overweight), gastric bypass surgery is another option for losing weight. This weight-reduction surgery, known generally as bariatric surgery, changes the anatomy of the digestive system to limit the amount of food a person can eat and digest. According to the 2004 *National Geographic* article "Why Are We So Fat?" 103,200 gastric bypass surgeries were performed in 2003, even though the failure rate of such surgeries looms at around 15 percent.

Medicare budget. Among the poor and disabled covered by Medicaid, 30 percent were obese, according to the 2004 study; the annual health-care costs they incurred approached $21 billion, or approximately 11 percent of Medicaid health spending. In total, obese patients receiving Medicare or Medicaid benefits accounted for 49 percent of the total obesity-related health expenditures in the United States. The other 51 percent of costs fell not just on private insurers, but also on individuals (studies indicate that obese Americans can expect to pay significantly more than their normal-weight counterparts for health care—some 36 percent more for those in the age group 18–36, for example). Obese Americans incur higher costs, on average, for more doctor's office visits, outpatient and inpatient hospital care, and prescription drugs—and these costs have been rising in recent years. If the trends continue, all Americans are likely to pay more and more in medical insurance premiums, co-payments, and other expenses related to health care.

Obesity is not only about economic costs, however. It is also about the human cost in misery and grief. Too many Americans who eat too much and exercise too little die too soon.

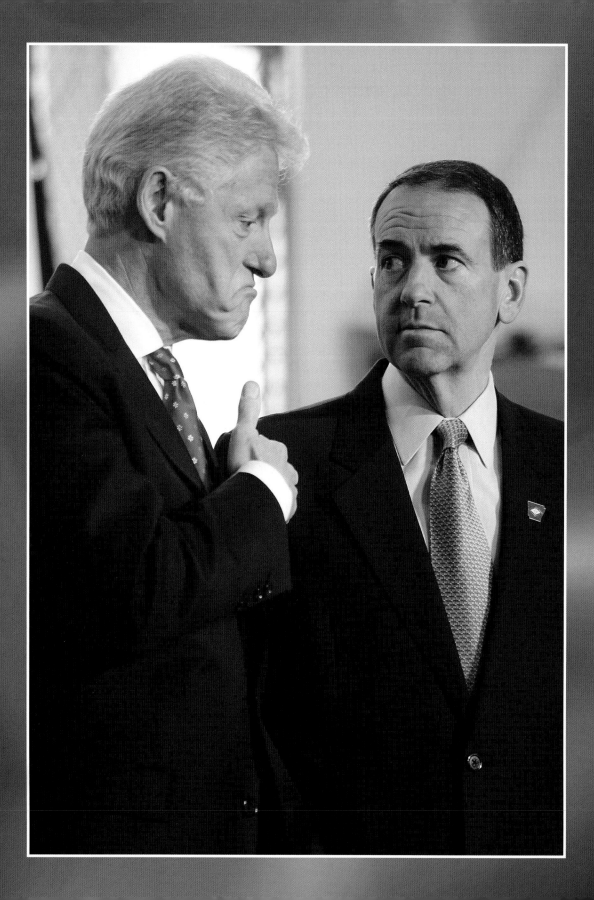

THE POLITICS OF OBESITY

4

The obesity crisis does not fall within the purview of the health-care system only. The federal government has stepped up its efforts to combat obesity, and states too have entered the fray—though many are discovering that the costs of treating obesity may soon overwhelm state health budgets and lead to reductions in other spending. Many insurance and health-care experts now believe that the problem of obesity costs states almost as much as tobacco-related diseases.

On March 12, 2004, President George W. Bush committed his administration to the war on obesity. Citing recent reports published by the Centers for Disease Control and Prevention, Bush promised to help end "poor diet and physical inactivity." Echoing the president, Surgeon General Richard Carmona stated, "I refuse to accept the spread of obesity. . . . I am committed to advancing the prevention agenda. . . . It will take all of us working together to find the solution to this growing problem."

Good intentions notwithstanding, obesity has emerged as a hot-button political issue. Few

(Opposite) Politicians weigh in on obesity: Former president Bill Clinton (left) and Arkansas governor Mike Huckabee confer during an event to publicize the launch of a 10-year initiative to combat the "national epidemic" of childhood obesity, May 3, 2005.

oppose encouraging Americans to live healthier lives, but critics of government programs wonder to what degree the government should invade the privacy of its citizens in that quest. On one hand, liberals maintain that there is a need to urge the government to regulate a food industry that they believe manipulates the public into eating fatty foods with little or no nutritional value. On the other hand, conservatives argue that individuals must be free to make their own choices, but must at the same time take responsibility for their actions and accept the consequences. An Associated Press story that appeared in 2003 summed up the controversy this way:

> The left's [liberal] view is that the food industry and advertisers are big bullies that practically force-feed people with gimmicks and high-calorie treats. They say Ronald McDonald is the cousin of Joe Camel.
>
> The right's [conservative] argument has been dubbed: You're fat, your fault. They say people can make their own choices about food and exercise.

The debate has begun to influence public policy, in the form of proposals for a junk-food tax and for limits on food advertising, in the demand for more detailed food labeling, and in lawsuits against food manufacturers and fast-food restaurant chains. Several states are considering imposing limits on sweets sold in schools; some are debating whether to force chain restaurants to list nutrition information on menus. While debate rages, the fact remains that Americans are getting fatter and sicker.

OBESITY ON CAPITOL HILL

By the beginning of the 21st century, then, obesity was no longer a private health concern but also a political issue. Like the president, members of Congress saw the need to promote a healthier way of life for all Americans. They advocated nutrition education programs for schoolchildren and initiatives to promote greater physical activity among citizens of all ages; they also pushed government programs and agencies (including Medicare, Medicaid, and the Social Security Administration) to redefine obesity.

Taking leading roles in the federal government's campaign against obesity have been the Food and Drug Administration (FDA) and the U.S. Department of Agriculture (USDA). In March 2004 a special FDA task force called the Obesity Working Group developed a number of proposals to address the problem. These included emphasizing all available treatment and medication therapies, enforcing accurate descriptions of serving sizes on all packaged and prepared foods, and asking the restaurant industry to voluntarily provide nutritional information about meals. The task force also advocated stepping up education programs about healthy eating, increasing research on obesity and related health concerns, and labeling food more accurately by defining such terms as "reduced calorie" and "low calorie." In 2005 the USDA introduced a new food pyramid that updated the recommended daily portions of foods from various food groups and more clearly identified those that promoted good nutrition and good health.

Among the obesity-related legislation recently introduced in Congress was the 2004 Prevention of Childhood Obesity Act. The act would, among other provisions, require elementary and secondary schools receiving federal aid to ban vending machines selling soda, candy, and other snacks of low nutritional value; provide grants for communities and schools to implement physical-activity programs for kids; and establish funding for after-school programs aimed at changing behavior that puts children at risk for obesity. Another program was aimed at creating a new federal commission on obesity treatment and prevention to work with local organizations through grants at the state and local levels; its proposed annual budget totaled $430 million.

The new food pyramid, released in April 2005, spotlights the importance of a balanced diet—as well as regular exercise.

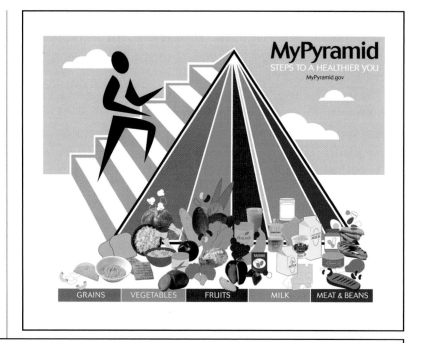

MyPyramid
STEPS TO A HEALTHIER YOU
MyPyramid.gov

| GRAINS | VEGETABLES | FRUITS | MILK | MEAT & BEANS |

GRAINS Make half your grains whole	VEGETABLES Vary your veggies	FRUITS Focus on fruits	MILK Get your calcium-rich foods	MEAT & BEANS Go lean with protein
Eat at least 3 oz. of whole-grain cereals, breads, crackers, rice, or pasta every day 1 oz. is about 1 slice of bread, about 1 cup of breakfast cereal, or ½ cup of cooked rice, cereal, or pasta	Eat more dark-green veggies like broccoli, spinach, and other dark leafy greens Eat more orange vegetables like carrots and sweetpotatoes Eat more dry beans and peas like pinto beans, kidney beans, and lentils	Eat a variety of fruit Choose fresh, frozen, canned, or dried fruit Go easy on fruit juices	Go low-fat or fat-free when you choose milk, yogurt, and other milk products If you don't or can't consume milk, choose lactose-free products or other calcium sources such as fortified foods and beverages	Choose low-fat or lean meats and poultry Bake it, broil it, or grill it Vary your protein routine — choose more fish, beans, peas, nuts, and seeds

For a 2,000-calorie diet, you need the amounts below from each food group. To find the amounts that are right for you, go to MyPyramid.gov.

| Eat 6 oz. every day | Eat 2½ cups every day | Eat 2 cups every day | Get 3 cups every day;
for kids aged 2 to 8, it's 2 | Eat 5½ oz. every day |

Find your balance between food and physical activity
- Be sure to stay within your daily calorie needs.
- Be physically active for at least 30 minutes most days of the week.
- About 60 minutes a day of physical activity may be needed to prevent weight gain.
- For sustaining weight loss, at least 60 to 90 minutes a day of physical activity may be required.
- Children and teenagers should be physically active for 60 minutes every day, or most days.

Know the limits on fats, sugars, and salt (sodium)
- Make most of your fat sources from fish, nuts, and vegetable oils.
- Limit solid fats like butter, stick margarine, shortening, and lard, as well as foods that contain these.
- Check the Nutrition Facts label to keep saturated fats, trans fats, and sodium low.
- Choose food and beverages low in added sugars. Added sugars contribute calories with few, if any, nutrients.

MyPyramid.gov
STEPS TO A HEALTHIER YOU

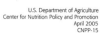

U.S. Department of Agriculture
Center for Nutrition Policy and Promotion
April 2005
CNPP-15

USDA

In the meantime, states such as Arkansas, Kansas, and Illinois have passed similar measures to create their own state commissions and programs for children.

The Workforce Health Improvement Program (WHIP), introduced into the Senate in 2005, proposed that employers be allowed to take a tax deduction for the cost of health-club memberships for their employees. Another resolution asked that private health insurance companies reward prevention rather than continuing to pay out billions to cover the costs of treatment. Along the same lines, the YMCA Healthy Teen Act proposed to teach teenagers how to live healthier lives and thereby to prevent unhealthy and risky behaviors later on. Similar ideas under consideration include offering better education for teenagers about eating disorders and obesity.

STATE AND LOCAL LEGISLATION

As mentioned, many states and cities also have begun to consider laws of their own. As of 2005, more than 142 new proposals were under consideration or had been passed in various state legislatures. In 2003 New York State assemblyman Felix Ortiz proposed a bill to institute a one-cent tax on all junk food, video games, and

PYRAMID FOR LIFE

On April 11, 2005, the federal government unveiled a revised food pyramid that emphasized eating a variety of foods and underscored the importance of physical activity. Known as the Food Guidance System, the new pyramid sports colorful stripes for each food group from tip to base, rather than the horizontal categories of the former version. It also includes a staircase along one side as a reminder to sedentary Americans to be more active. The pyramid is based on the 2005 U.S. dietary guidelines, which stress the importance of fruits, vegetables, whole grains, and healthful fat, including nuts and olive oil. It also emphasizes limiting the intake of sugar, saturated fat, and trans-fatty acids, which are often found in junk foods and fast foods.

television commercials. Also known as the "couch potato tax," the measure was intended to fund physical and nutrition education programs in schools. In addition to Ortiz's proposal, legislation was introduced in New York that would institute a $500 tax credit for individuals who bought exercise equipment or joined a health club. As of mid-2005, that measure—called the New York Fitness Income Tax Credit, or NY-FIT—and Ortiz's proposal were both pending.

With the California Childhood Obesity Prevention Act, introduced in 2003 and passed into law, certain nutrition standards are required for all beverages sold to students in California's elementary, middle, and junior high schools. Beginning in July 2004, only certain beverages, such as water, milk, 100 percent fruit juices, and fruit-based drinks with no less than 50 percent fruit juice and no added sweeteners, could be sold in schools.

On the local level, Mayor Kwame Kilpatrick of Detroit proposed in May 2005 a two-cent tax on fast food in addition to the six-cent sales tax on all restaurant meals. To many it seemed an appropriate tax, since Detroit ranked as the nation's fattest city in 2005. The Detroit tax would be the first to target fast-food outlets, according to the National Restaurant Association, and would apply to everything sold, including salads.

Other local initiatives included the Tweens Nutrition and Fitness Coalition, organized in Lexington, Kentucky, during the summer of 2004. Hundreds of children between the ages of 7 and 14 increased their physical activity throughout the summer. To monitor progress, each child was given a scorecard with 24 blank squares. Every time a child went to a specified site, such as a swimming pool, martial arts class, or bowling alley, his or her card was stamped. Parents also awarded stamps each time their child or children engaged in some sort of physical activity for an hour. Other incentives to participate were the special rewards that the coalition offered, such as free admission to sports clinics.

If a child completely filled his or her scorecard by a specified date, he or she was eligible for a Grand Celebration prize. Not only did the program generate enthusiasm among children, it also got parents and local businesses involved in supporting physical activities for youth.

Also beginning in 2004, many local schools and communities formed partnerships with CIGNA, an insurance and health-benefits company, to organize education programs and to promote physical fitness and good nutrition. The company already had adopted a similar program for the children of its employees and hoped by 2005 to make the program available to all CIGNA clients.

WHOSE BUSINESS IS IT, ANYWAY?

Even as government agencies, legislatures, Congress, and the White House are taking a more active role in

At this camp located in Pennsylvania's Pocono Mountains, overweight adolescents learn good nutrition and exercise habits.

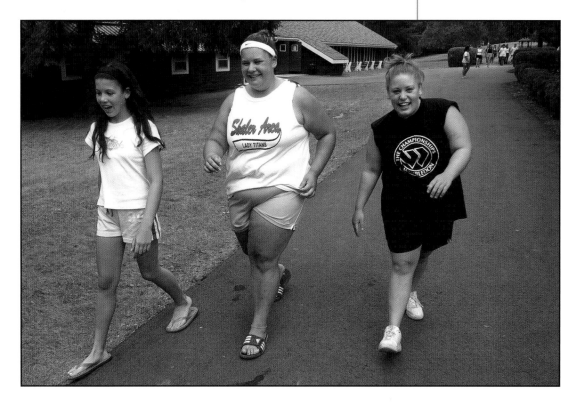

combating obesity, another debate is under way. Specifically, many Americans are now asking just how large a role the government should take when it comes to fighting obesity. There are compelling arguments for and against government intervention in the issue.

If numbers are any indication, government participation in the war on obesity is not entirely welcome. A poll conducted in the summer of 2003 by Harvard Forums on Health showed Americans evenly divided on the question of government intervention in a matter of personal health. Of the 1,002 queried, 48 percent said that obesity is a private concern and a personal responsibility; according to these respondents, it is up to individuals to take care of their own weight and health. Forty-seven percent of the respondents disagreed, stating that obesity is a public health issue requiring government intervention. At the same time, however, consensus was clear in certain areas: 75 percent supported government education campaigns, while 81 percent believed the government should create more parks or recreation areas to encourage Americans to be more active. Yet when asked if they supported a special tax on junk food, 59 percent said no.

The Harvard poll found overwhelming support for the expansion of health and physical education programs for children and the creation of more nutritious lunch programs. Many of those polled also supported the general involvement of schools in fighting childhood obesity.

The respondents, however, were unsure how the government ought to pay for such initiatives. Although 76 percent said they were willing to pay higher taxes to fund anti-obesity programs for children, many put limits on their generosity. Only 42 percent stated that they would be willing to pay more than $100 a year.

Respondents to the Harvard poll also saw a role for the private sector to play in fighting obesity. Three in four said that health-care providers should assume a major role in addressing the problem of overweight Americans. In addition, 62 percent agreed that restaurants should be required to list nutrition information on their menus.

SOCIAL ENGINEERING AND THE GOVERNMENT

If many Americans are wary of aggressive government intervention in issues such as obesity, labeling such intervention social engineering, many others believe government action is quite appropriate in dealing with matters that affect the health of the public. Implicitly, these proponents of social engineering believe that it is among the most important responsibilities of government to save the American people from themselves, whether it be from their poor eating habits, inadequate exercise, unsafe sexual practices, dangerous products, smoking, drinking, or other risky behaviors. It is also the role of government, they believe, to instill new and better attitudes in the younger generation, to prevent the recurrence of problems in the future. Such methods, activists reassure the public, will ultimately save money and lives.

The champions of government intervention thus call on the government to institute fundamental changes in the way Americans eat and live. Not only should the government regulate different types of foods, they argue, but it must also, for example, study how cities can be redesigned in order to promote greater physical activity. Furthermore, activists insist, the government ought to prohibit on school grounds the marketing and sale of food products that are nutritionally unsound and ban all fast foods, snack foods, and soft drinks from school vending machines and lunch menus. Some even support laws, similar to those governing alcoholic beverages, to prohibit the sale of fast food within a certain distance of school grounds. But the most committed activists would not stop there. In their view, state legislatures that refused to support

Lifestyle choices like exercising regularly, eating nutritious foods, and maintaining a good weight confer health benefits on the individual—and may benefit society in the form of increased worker productivity and reduced health-care expenditures. Still, critics say, individuals should be free to decide how they want to live, without government efforts to "save" them from their own bad choices.

this ambitious agenda should be penalized through litigation, fines, or the withholding of federal funds. To pay for such extensive anti-obesity programs, the advocates of government intervention suggest a combination of taxes, subsidies, and regulatory fees.

Opponents of extensive government involvement in combating obesity couldn't disagree more with this agenda. The anti-obesity activists, they say, are merely frightened and manipulative elitists who advocate government intervention because they don't trust ordinary people to make sensible and rational decisions on their own. "What is next after food?" one opponent of government interference wondered. "Will they start telling us how many push-ups to do every day?"

Should Americans be free (as long as their behavior doesn't impinge on the freedom of others) to live a lifestyle of their choosing, even if that lifestyle harms them? Or does government's responsibility to promote and protect public health justify intervention to discourage—if necessary by punitive measures such as taxes—behavior that might lead to disease, injury, or death? Those questions reflect the deep philosophical divide in the debate over obesity and public policy.

CHEESEBURGER AND FRIES GO TO COURT

One trend for which Americans show little support is the growing number of obesity lawsuits against the fast-food industry. The lawsuit trend began in July 2002, when a 56-year-old obese man unsuccessfully sued McDonald's, Burger King, Kentucky Fried Chicken, and

Wendy's, charging that their food had caused his obesity. This was quickly followed by a class-action lawsuit, in which two Bronx teenagers claimed that McDonald's used false advertising and that the chain's food made them fat and contributed to their health problems. The lawyers for the two teenagers also asserted that unknown ingredients and processing made foods such as french fries, Chicken McNuggets, and Filet-O-Fish sandwiches damaging to their clients', and the general public's, health. The federal judge hearing the case was not sympathetic to these arguments. In his decision throwing out the lawsuit, handed down in September 2004, the judge stated, "If a person knows or should know that eating copious orders of super-sized McDonald's products is unhealthy and may result in weight gain . . . it is not the place of the law to protect them from their own excesses."

Most Americans agreed. In a July 2003 Gallup poll, the public voiced its growing impatience with lawsuits blaming the fast-food industry for obesity and failing to hold individuals accountable for their own conduct. The poll found that 42 percent of Americans believed that the fast-food industry was "not at all responsible" for the obesity problems in the country. An additional 25 percent felt the fast-food industry was "not too responsible" for Americans' obesity. Further, the poll found that approximately 9 out of 10 Americans (89 percent) opposed holding the fast-food industry legally responsible for the diet and health-related problems of people who chose to eat fast food on a regular basis. Fifty-three percent of those polled knew that fast food was not good for people to eat on a regular basis. However, those with a college education and above-average incomes were more likely to respond critically to the nutritional content of fast foods.

Despite opinions such as those recorded in the Gallup poll and despite court defeats, trial lawyers—

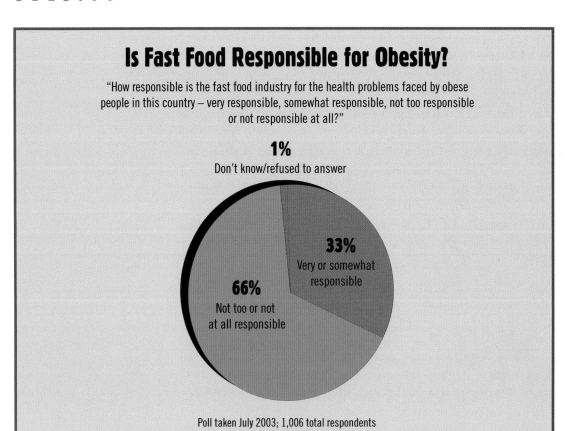

Is Fast Food Responsible for Obesity?

"How responsible is the fast food industry for the health problems faced by obese people in this country – very responsible, somewhat responsible, not too responsible or not responsible at all?"

1%
Don't know/refused to answer

33%
Very or somewhat responsible

66%
Not too or not at all responsible

Poll taken July 2003; 1,006 total respondents
Source: The Gallup Organization

perhaps sensing the potential for the kind of multibillion-dollar settlement the tobacco industry paid—continue to pursue a growing number of targets in the fast-food and junk-food industries. Lawsuits have been aimed at popular snacks such as Oreo cookies, as well as the operators of school vending machines. Lawyers have even considered suing doctors, parents, and school boards for contributing to, or failing to prevent, obesity in the children under their care.

However, with the federal passage of the so-called Cheeseburger Bill in March 2004, the number of lawsuits against food companies has been limited severely. Many states have followed the federal government's lead: by July 2004, a total of 12 states had enacted laws that protected restaurants and food producers from frivolous lawsuits.

Personal responsibility and individual freedom remain important values to most Americans. For a small yet vocal minority, however, the perception that an obesity crisis looms is reason to give government greater control over how Americans should eat. Whether the answer is greater personal responsibility or more regulatory measures enacted by the government, the debate continues.

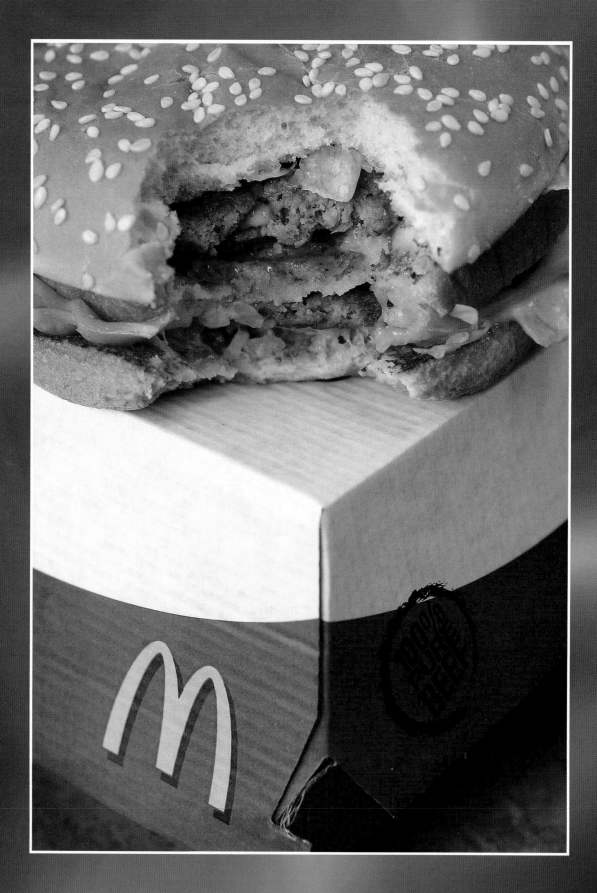

SUPERSIZING AND SLENDERIZING: PROFITING FROM OBESITY

5

When foreigners are asked to describe the United States, one adjective that invariably comes to mind is *big*. The United States is a big country. Even in this time of rising gasoline prices, Americans like to drive in big cars. They live in big houses. They make big deals. Physically, Americans are also big. They have, in fact, grown much taller and heavier during the last 200 years.

Americans also eat big. They are bombarded with advertisements telling them that a robust appetite is good and that it's okay to eat and drink too much. There are, after all, pharmacies stocked with medications to soothe indigestion, calm heartburn, and cure headaches. So, go ahead and live a little. Americans have carried

(Opposite) Fast food, like this McDonald's Big Mac, tends to be high in fat, high in calories, and high in sodium. Still, Americans love burgers and french fries and soda—and, it seems, the bigger the meal, the better.

on a long love affair with all-you-can-eat buffets, "supersized" portions, and "mega" soft drinks. Even the names of many fast-food offerings suggest their mammoth proportions: McDonald's Big Mac and Quarter Pounder, Burger King's Whopper, 7-11's Super Slurp, Wendy's Biggie Fries and Biggie Drink, Hardee's Monster Burger.

Besides being big eaters, Americans benefit from one of the most efficient food industries in the world. National Public Radio reported, in a 1999 story, that the American food industry produces more than a trillion calories a day. That breaks down to approximately 3,800 calories for every man, woman, and child in the United States, or 1,300 calories more than the recommended daily maximum intake of 2,500 for men (the recommended maximum for women is about 2,000 calories). Those excess calories, one physician noted, "end up going to waste or to the waist." Even if a person consumed only 100 extra calories per day, he or she would on average gain one pound per month.

The food industry is eager to sell as many calories to the American people as possible. Economic survival depends on it. Operating with huge advertising budgets, the food industry inundates Americans with television, radio, and print ads.

BARGAIN OR BALANCE?

In a 2002 press release from the Center for Science in the Public Interest (CSPI), Margo Wootan, director of nutrition policy for the organization, stated: "Americans are constantly induced to spend a little more money to get a lot more food. Getting more for your money is ingrained in the American psyche. But bigger is rarely better when it comes to food."

Wootan was responding to a report titled "From Wallet to Waistline: The Hidden Costs of Super Sizing," compiled by the National Alliance for Nutrition and Activity (NANA), a coalition of more than 225 national, state, and local health organizations. In the report, NANA compared prices, calories, and amount of saturated fat in differently sized foods from a variety of sources, including fast-food chains, convenience stores, ice cream parlors, coffee shops, and movie theaters. NANA's findings revealed troubling patterns in food marketing and sales techniques, which, it said, are having an unhealthy influence on Americans' eating habits. According to the report:

> Upgrading from a 3-ounce Minibon to a Classic Cinnabon costs only 24% more, yet delivers 123% more calories and provides almost three-quarters of a day's worth of . . . saturated fat. . . . Switching from 7-Eleven's Gulp to a Double Gulp costs 42% more, but provides 300% more calories. . . . It costs 8 cents more to purchase a McDonald's Quarter Pounder with Cheese, small French fries, and small Coke (890 calories) than it costs to buy the Quarter Pounder with Cheese large Extra Value Meal, which comes with a large fries and large Coke (1,380 calories). . . . A 23% increase in price [for movie theater popcorn] provides 125% more calories.

To the CSPI, bargain meals are not exactly bargains when it comes to healthy eating. Similarly, in the minds of nutritionists and doctors, the practice of selling tasty but high-fat, high-calorie food at low prices should set off alarms for consumers. From the perspective of psychology professor Kelly D. Brownell, the practice is downright sinister. Brownell regards food bargains as "consumer exploitation" because "people have biological vulnerabilities that promote overeating when large portions are available, a strong desire for value, and the capacity to be persuaded by advertising."

PACKAGING GLUTTONY

The long road to supersizing started with one small step. During the 1970s, plagued by high food prices and double-digit inflation, Americans were struggling to save money. David Wallerstein, an executive director at McDonald's Corporation, saw both a problem and an opportunity in American frugality. Wallerstein under-stood that he had to overcome more than a temporary economic slowdown that made people wary about spending money. He also had to overcome a cultural belief of long standing: gluttony was bad; it was, in fact, counted among the seven deadly sins.

Almost a decade earlier, as an executive in the movie theater business, Wallerstein had grappled with a similar problem. He realized that money was made not simply from selling movie tickets but also from marketing concessions. He tried a number of different approaches to increase concession sales, but nothing generated additional profits. In his book *Fat Land*, Greg Critser described what happened next:

> Thinking about it one night, [Wallerstein] had a realiza-tion: People did not want to buy two boxes of popcorn no matter what. They didn't want to be seen eating two boxes of popcorn. It looked . . . piggish. . . . Perhaps he could get more people to spend a little more on popcorn if he made the boxes bigger and increased the price only a little.

The following week, Wallerstein put his theory to the test, and the results exceeded even his expectations. Sales increased and profits soared. Not only did the sale of popcorn rise, but so did sales of candy and soda.

A decade later, Wallerstein pitched this approach to Ray Kroc, the founder of McDonald's. At the time, most customers were only buying burgers and sodas, even though it was clear that people also liked the taste of McDonald's french fries. Wallerstein attributed the low french fry sales to two factors: first, customers were unwilling to pay the extra cost, and second, they didn't want to appear gluttonous by ordering multiple food items. Wallerstein believed that the second factor could be overcome if customers thought they were get-ting a good deal, so he suggested that McDonald's begin to sell larger bags of fries at a cheaper price. This, he insisted, would make it very difficult for people to resist giving in to their desire to buy the fries. At first, Kroc was reluctant to follow Wallerstein's advice, fearing the scheme would cost him money. But as sales continued to lag, he relented. In just a few months, sales of french fries at McDonald's restaurants throughout the United States increased dramatically. Wallerstein's hunch had paid off. It marked the beginning of "supersizing."

Over the next decade, a number of fast-food chains took advantage of the low prices for meat, sugar, bread, and cheese to initiate some variation of supersizing. Customers soon were offered a variety of different meal combinations while still enjoying the option of increasing the size of their portions at a comparatively low cost. Americans were eating greater quantities of food than ever before, dramatically increasing their daily caloric

The roots of the fast-food companies' successful "supersizing" campaigns can be traced to an insight that movie theater executive David Wallerstein had in the 1960s. If he offered patrons a lot more popcorn for only a little more money, Wallerstein realized, they would buy more.

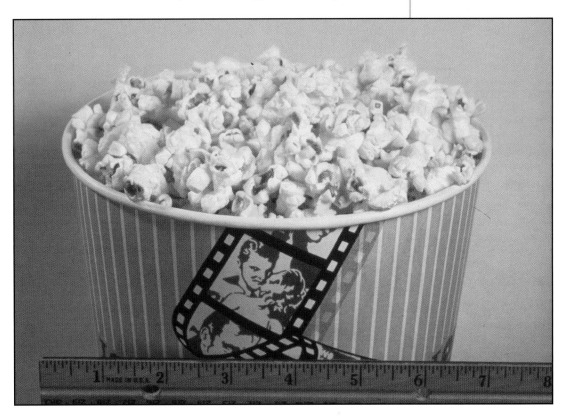

intake and ingesting unhealthful amounts of fat, sugar, salt, and chemical preservatives. For many dietitians, these developments constituted a nutritional nightmare. Those consumers who liked the convenience and flavor of fast food, however, were getting more value for their money, and that was a bottom line that satisfied every-one except those concerned about obesity and health.

FAST-FOOD NATION

During the last three decades, Americans have developed their taste for fast food. In 1972 they spent $3 billion a year on fast food. By 2005 that figure had risen to more than $110 billion.

Fast food is now undeniably a daily part of American life. Consider that each day one in every four Americans visits a fast-food restaurant. The most profitable chain, McDonald's, feeds more than 46 million Americans—more than the entire population of Spain—daily. And the marketing department at the McDonald's Corporation isn't satisfied; the goal is to serve every McDonald's customer 20 times a month.

Fast food provides one-third of many diners' daily caloric intake; however, fast-food meals include almost no milk, fruit, or nonstarchy vegetables, all of which are key ingredients in a healthy, balanced diet. As a person's frequency of fast-food consumption increases, the intake of important minerals and vitamins—such as vitamins A and C, beta-carotenes, calcium, phosphorus, and magnesium—decreases markedly.

Over time, too, the total calories in typical fast-food meals have grown. At McDonald's, a regular serving of fries originally was 200 calories. Today, it is 610. The basic meal of a hamburger, small french fries, and soft drink was a modest 590 calories. Today, a typical super-sized meal provides a whopping 1,550 calories, which constitutes almost 78 percent of the recommended maximum daily caloric intake for women, and 62 percent of the recommended daily maximum for men. Even as some chains are starting to build up leaner and healthier menu offerings, the notion of a big sandwich or burger shows no sign of fading away. In 2004, for example, Hardee's unveiled its Monster Burger, consisting of two 1/3-pound slabs of Angus beef, four strips of bacon, three slices of American cheese, and mayonnaise—all on a buttered, sesame-seed bun. The burger alone provides 1,420 calories; with fries and a soft drink added, the total number of calories is nearly equal to the daily caloric needs for even the most active adults.

A NORMAL PORTION?

Portions served by fast-food chains and other restaurants are far larger than the USDA-recommended serving sizes for most foods. Food costs for restaurants are relatively low (compared with the costs of rent and labor), so for restaurant owners it makes sense to offer larger portions, which make customers feel that they are getting the most for their money.

As Americans eat out more frequently, they become accustomed to oversized portions and think that these portions are normal. The high caloric content of these larger servings leads to weight gain for customers who eat out frequently, and this, in turn, has led to other, more serious health problems. Unfortunately, fast-food chains and restaurants do not consistently alert customers to the hazardously high calorie and fat content of the food they serve.

While fast-food chains may have started the trend, more traditional restaurants and even grocery stores have followed suit by enlarging their portions. Muffins, for example, are typically 333 percent larger than the USDA recommends; a normal serving of pasta is 480 percent bigger. Typical bagels now weigh between four and seven ounces, when one ounce is defined as a single grain serving. Packaged and processed foods also fuel this trend. Even cookbooks are using recipes that specify fewer servings for the same amounts of ingredients, meaning portions are expected to be larger.

Over time, people became used to eating larger servings. In a 2001 study conducted at Penn State University, a group of male and female volunteers were served lunch on four different occasions. At each session, the size of the entrée was increased, from 500 grams to 625, then to 750, and finally to 1,000 grams. By the end of the study, which spanned a month, the volunteers were eating the larger amounts without difficulty. The researchers' conclusion was unsettling: hunger and the capacity to consume grew to accommodate the larger servings.

Today, the word *supersizing* has become commonplace. Yet, its appeal remains largely undiminished. As marketing consultant Irma Zall pointed out, "Bigness is addictive because it is about power." Even if, for example, few teenage boys can finish a 64-ounce Double Gulp, Zall says that "it's empowering to hold one in your hand." Size matters, and evidently it matters a great deal to many Americans. Although they may feel a sense of power at their ability to consume larger portions, Americans have ironically acquiesced in becoming a fast-food nation, complacently accepting the creed that gluttony is good and ignoring what processed foods are doing to their bodies and their health.

Where prepared food is concerned, Americans have gotten used to very large portions. A typical slice of pizza is likely to comprise what nutritionists would define as two (or even three) normal servings.

PROFITS AND (WEIGHT) LOSSES

If many companies have reaped healthy profits by providing Americans the nutritionally questionable and oversized meals they crave, many other companies have found that helping Americans lose the weight they put on through such bad eating habits is also a lucrative business. Americans spend more than $30 billion each year seeking an antidote to obesity. The diet industry offers everything from books to tapes, from "lite" foods to low-cal beverages, from exercise regimens to commercial weight-loss programs. There are also a number of crash-diet plans that promise consumers rapid weight loss if they drink specially formulated drinks or take weight-loss pills.

Diets have been around at least since the 1830s, when Sylvester Graham, who invented the Graham cracker as an alternative to meat, preached against the sin of gluttony and urged his audiences to curb their appetites for both food and sex. Later, in the mid-1960s, diets became a national mania. That's because being fat was, for the first time, considered a medical problem, and thinness, especially for women, became the ideal of beauty. Weight loss measures grew extreme by the 1970s, with high-protein diets such as Robert Linn's liquid diet and the Complete Scarsdale Diet. By the end of that decade, there were more than a hundred different diet programs, most of them designed or endorsed by doctors; those numbers would triple by the mid-1980s. Today, there are literally thousands of diet plans to choose from.

But the weight-loss industry is by no means confined to diet plans. Pharmaceutical companies have developed a succession of drugs to curb appetite and, more recently, lower cholesterol. Weight Watchers, an organization that promotes a comprehensive approach to diet and nutrition, conducts support classes and offers its own line of healthful food products.

The American weight-loss industry today is huge, fluid, and dynamic. No single organization—indeed, no single approach—dominates; rather, there are a host of companies and individuals offering various products, services, and philosophies to those wishing to trim down. Yet there is no denying the fact that, as a whole, the weight-loss industry is big business. Sales of weight-loss products came to almost $48.6 billion in

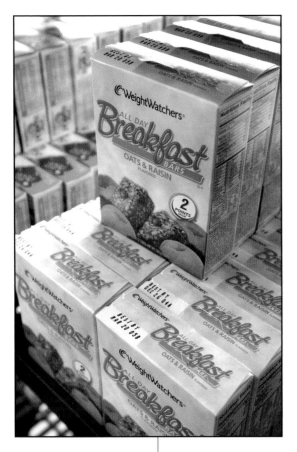

As Americans have packed on the pounds, the weight loss industry has become big business. Seen here are boxes of Weight Watchers breakfast bars.

2005, and by 2008 that number was expected to grow to nearly $61 billion. It seems certain that steady demand for weight-loss services—whether delivered via the Internet, a local weight-loss center, a family physician, a health club, a hospital, or a pill—will continue as long as obesity rates remain high.

LOW-FAT, LOW-CARB

Not everyone who is overweight or obese wants to follow a supervised weight-loss plan. Many simply do not want to go to a hospital, clinic, or weight-loss center. Others cannot afford the cost of such programs. Instead, many Americans choose to go it alone, by following an unstructured, flexible, and affordable program. The weight-loss industry has responded with a whole host of products designed for the individual dieter.

Every decade some new diet or medical advice grips Americans. Two of the most recent were low-fat diets, popular during the 1980s and 1990s, and low-carb diets, which have been around in some form or another since the 1970s. In each case, individuals cut the dietary culprit—either fat or carbohydrates—from their diets in order to lose weight.

In response to the popularity of the low-fat diet, more than 3,000 new low-fat food products had been introduced to American consumers by the 1990s. And yet, over the course of the decade, the number of overweight Americans increased by 15 percent, according to the National Center for Health Statistics, and the average American man's waist size increased by an inch and a half. The low-fat foods became a license to indulge, as dieters gobbled up low-fat ice creams, cakes, and brownies. Simply put, because the foods were labeled "low-fat," Americans assumed they were low in everything else too. But the reality was that in order to make low-fat foods taste palatable, manufacturers had to load them up with extra sugar. The fat content was lower, but the calories remained the same, so instead of losing extra pounds, many Americans actually gained weight. By the late 1990s it was clear that the low-fat diets were not working, and groups such as the USDA and the American Dietetic Association (ADA) began moderating their recommendations.

By the 1990s, the low-fat diet was losing ground to the low-carb diet, the most prominent proponent of which was an American physician named Robert Atkins. The Atkins diet actually encouraged people to eat fatty foods such as red meat, butter, eggs, and bacon. What low-carb dieters had to avoid were foods filled with carbohydrates, such as grains, fruits, juices, and sweets. Food manufacturers quickly responded to the fad. Among their offerings were snacks allowing low-carb dieters to indulge a sweet tooth, such as cookies, cakes, and candy that had been reformulated to take out the harmful sugars and other ingredients. Even low-carb soft drinks and beers were marketed. Unfortunately, many low-carb dieters—and low-fat dieters, for that matter—ended up forgoing foods and nutrients that are a vital source of energy and nutrition in a healthy diet.

Overall, diets of any kind tend to work very poorly; most people can lose only about 10 percent of their body weight, and most will gain back their lost weight over time. The proliferation of best-selling diet books published in the past five years is an ironic twist to the health concerns among overweight Americans striving to lose weight. These popular diets typically offer

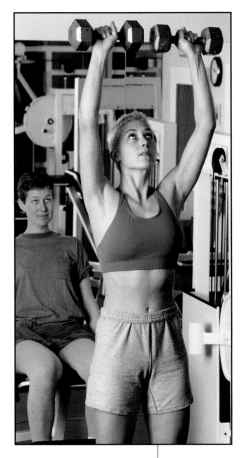

Various studies have shown that many American women are insecure about their own body images. But overweight women are less likely than their thin or normal-weight counterparts to exercise. Instead they tend to rely on diet pills and fad diets, which offer generally low rates of long-term success in weight loss.

dieters empty promises, such as rapid weight loss, increased energy level, and absence of hunger or food deprivation. But these diets typically put severe limitations on what can and cannot be eaten, and many people quickly tire of eating the same things over and over again, increasing their chances of failure. In part because so many dieters fail to follow sound weight-loss practices, approximately 70 percent regain at least half of their lost weight within two years.

While the best way to lose weight is to eat fewer calories and to exercise, this no-nonsense approach has found few takers. In 2005 the Centers for Disease Control and Prevention reported that only 17.5 percent of dieters try to consume fewer calories and increase their physical activity; approximately one in four dieters eats the recommended five servings of fruits and vegetables daily.

Many researchers and health-care professionals continue to stress the importance of exercise, no matter what a person weighs. Research has shown that the best indicator of overall health, for men and women, is not body weight but performance on a treadmill test. According to many health-care experts, it is better to be fat and fit than lean and unfit.

WOMEN AND SELF-IMAGE

In a 1998 survey of American women conducted by the Teresa and H. John Heinz III Foundation, 70 percent of overweight women, as opposed to 41 percent of thin women, reported that they liked their bodies less than they liked themselves. Comparing the attitudes and beliefs of overweight women aged 35 and over with their thin or normal-weight same-aged counterparts, the survey clearly found that many of the overweight women felt stigmatized because of their bodies. Specifically, more than one in four overweight women in the survey identified images of women in the media as making them feel worse about their bodies. Such negativity translates into a higher prevalence of unhealthy behaviors among overweight women. According to Barbara J. Moore, president of Shape Up America!, "This survey shows that the perpetuation of an unattainable body image for American women is not just demeaning, it's a public health threat." Even more troubling, the survey demonstrated differences in weight-management strategies employed by overweight versus thin and normal-weight women. Overweight women were less likely to exercise and more likely to use dieting and diet pills to manage their weight. In fact, overweight women more often reported unhealthy behaviors like eating disorders and use of appetite suppressants.

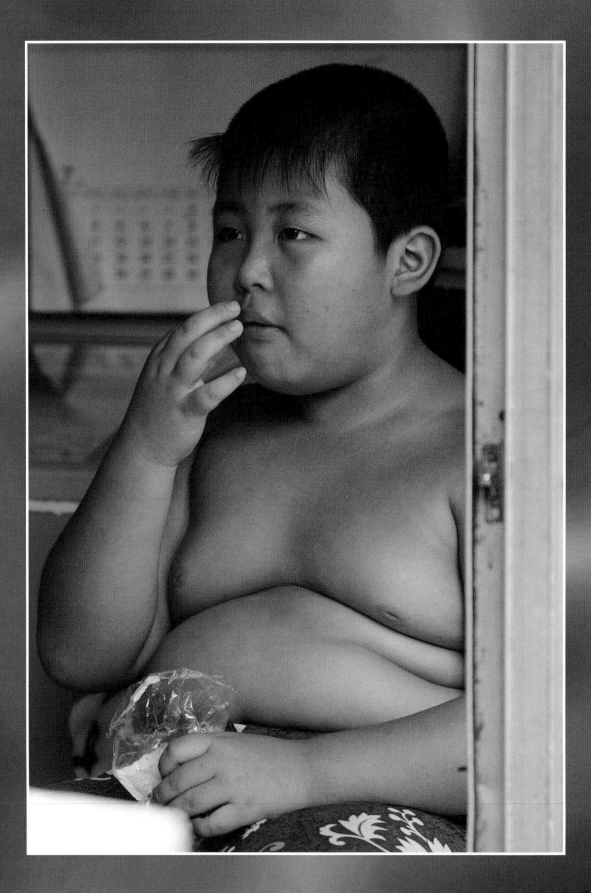

6

THE FUTURE IS NOW: CHILDREN & OBESITY

Nowhere is the problem of obesity more acute and painful than among America's children. As adults debate the cost and consequences of obesity, obese children move closer to a lifetime of health problems. The story of a girl named Alyssa, which is detailed in Dr. Sylvia Rimm's 2004 book, *Rescuing the Emotional Lives of Overweight Children*, is typical:

> Ever since I was a little kid, I was fat, and that made me feel different from other kids. Kids left me out of their groups. I had absolutely no one to play with on the playground; not a single friend. On Valentine's Day when the other kids got valentines . . . my valentine had an elephant on it. . . . I felt like an elephant.

While some obese children withdraw, separating themselves from their classmates, others deal with obesity using dark humor. *Sports Illustrated* writer Rick Reilly noted the following jump-rope rhyme, chanted by some obese grade-school girls:

Georgia, Texas

North Carolina!

According to government statistics, about 15 percent of American children and youth between the ages of 6 and 19 are overweight. Unfortunately, that puts them at higher risk for adult obesity, along with the range of adverse health consequences that accompany it.

I think I'm suff-ring

Acute angina!

OVERWEIGHT CHILDREN BY THE NUMBERS

Data compiled by the CDC's National Center for Health Statistics covering the years 1999–2002 show that 15 percent of Americans aged 6 to 11, and 15 percent aged 12 to 19, were overweight. This represents about 9 million American children and adolescents. A similar CDC survey taken between 1971 and 1974 showed that only 4 percent of children between the ages of 6 and 11, and only 6 percent of adolescents between the ages of 12 and 19, were overweight.

There is no one reason for the dramatic rise in the numbers of overweight American children. Fingers point at the fast-food industry, television advertising, school lunch programs, the lack of mandatory physical education courses, the greater reliance of families on prepared food, and even American children themselves, many of whom prefer to consume junk food, watch television, or play video games than to eat sensibly and participate in sports or similar activities.

Fast-food giants such as McDonald's and Burger King have reshaped the diets of many American children (as they have the diets of many American parents). The rise in fast-food consumption mirrors the rise of childhood and adolescent obesity. Between 1977 and 1995, the percentage of meals and snacks eaten at fast-food restaurants doubled. Because fast food is so high in sugar, fat, and calories, eating a regular diet of these foods can add pounds quickly. Along with consuming these high-sugar and high-fat foods, American children and adolescents also have increased their soft-drink consumption. Between 1977 and 1996, soda consumption among the 12–19 age group increased 75 percent for boys and 40 percent for girls.

Clearly, American children and adolescents love fast food. On a typical day, nearly one-third of Americans aged 4 to 19 consume fast food. Further, those who regularly eat fast food have been found to consume more total fat, more added sugars, more sugar-sweetened beverages, less fiber, fewer fruits, and fewer non-starchy vegetables than those who do not eat fast food. More than 60 percent of young people eat too much fat, and less than 20 percent eat the recommended daily serving of fruits and vegetables. Those meals add up; young people who eat fast food consume, on average, 187 additional calories a day, which could translate into an extra six pounds per year.

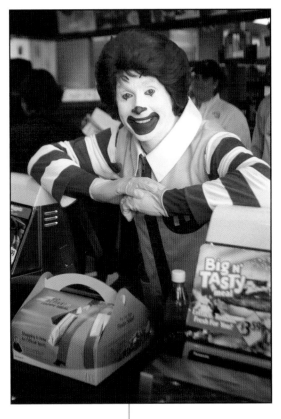

Ronald McDonald has helped attract several generations of young consumers to McDonald's restaurants. Other fast-food chains have created tie-ins with popular movies or cartoons in marketing campaigns aimed at kids.

CHILDHOOD FOR PROFIT

Beginning in the 1980s, fast-food restaurants and other food industries marketing snacks and prepared foods aggressively pursued young consumers. In doing so, they utilized a variety of tools, especially television, specially created characters and tie-ins with popular movies, and a greater commercial presence in schools. This marketing push came at a time when the number of two-income households was on the rise and parents on average spent more time away from the home. Many children had less supervision overall, and some were left to fend for themselves when dinnertime came. Even if they were at home by then, working parents might be too tired to fix meals, and so reliance on fast food and prepared foods increased.

Television, one of the food marketers' primary tools, is an obesity machine, both because of what it shows and because of the way it affects children's level of physical activity. Television gives advertisers a way to walk through the front door of any home and speak directly to children. The average American child watches 19 hours and 40 minutes of television per week, adding up to more than a thousand hours each year. That means annual exposure to thousands of commercials for junk food, fast food, soft drinks, sugar-laden cereals, and the like. Even when the television is not on, children and adolescents turn to other screens: computers and video games. Those aged 2 to 18 now spend an average of 38 hours per week sitting in front of some type of screen.

These hours spent in front of a television, computer, or game screen mean less time devoted to physical activity. And the more sedentary children are, the more likely they are to be overweight, now and in the future.

TEMPTATION THROUGH VARIOUS VENUES

Ask almost any parent about children and commercials, and they will explain that commercials for junk food and fast food are overwhelming for children. Growing evidence suggests that advertising to children can create a powerful desire for products. When junk-food companies realized the power that television marketing had over children, they invested heavily in it. In fact, sugared foods account for the largest portion of the television advertising addressed specifically to children.

Like parents, advertisers have long understood that young children are especially vulnerable to marketing ploys, in part because they do not realize they are being manipulated. Instead, children—particularly younger ones—are apt to see commercials as nothing more than information about foods they like to eat, games they want to play, or toys they wish to own. Saturday mornings are prime time when it comes to advertising geared toward children. In 1987, for instance, an average of 225 commercials were shown during peak

Saturday morning viewing hours. By the mid-1990s that number had jumped to 997. By 2005 it was estimated that children on average watched 40,000 commercials a year, two-thirds of which promoted foods that had limited or questionable nutritional value.

From the time McDonald's kicked off its first advertising campaign in 1967, company executives quickly realized that children constituted a large untapped audience. To reach these younger consumers, McDonald's created special children's meals such as the Happy Meal. Rival Burger King countered with the BK Kid's Meal. These meals generally included a hamburger or cheeseburger, fries, and a small soft drink. In time, most fast-food chains created a kid's menu.

To attract children more fully to their products, McDonald's, Burger King, Wendy's, and other fast-food companies have created elaborate marketing campaigns. Using familiar characters such as Disney's Winnie the Pooh or other popular characters from films such as *Star Wars*, *Shrek*, *SpongeBob SquarePants*, and *101 Dalmatians*, fast-food companies have combined food with toys or action figures. McDonald's even created its own characters, such as Ronald McDonald and the Hamburglar, to help sell its food to children.

Soft-drink companies also strenuously pitch their products to children and teens. Relying mostly on what is known as product placement, companies such as Coca-Cola and PepsiCo have been effective in marketing to children. By paying huge amounts of money to have their products featured in films aimed at children or to create tie-ins to films with popular characters such as Harry Potter, companies can dramatically increase sales. For instance, when the movie *E.T.* featured the lovable creature from outer space eating Reese's Pieces and liking them, sales rose 65 percent; Hershey, the maker of Reese's Pieces, had to put two factories on 24-hour production schedules to meet the increased

Lunchtime at a Chicago high school. The scene is typical: nearly 95 percent of American high schools, and about 60 percent of elementary schools, have vending machines that sell soda. Seven in 10 high schools also have vending machines that sell chocolate candy.

demand. Product placement is also a good way to establish brands in the minds of children. The objective, of course, is to create lifelong brand loyalty.

INVASION OF THE NUTRITION SNATCHERS

At one time, it was the responsibility of schools to teach students about the importance of good nutrition. Classes in health and hygiene stressed dietary needs and restrictions essential for students to stay healthy and strong. Home economics classes taught students how to cook nutritious meals. Physical education classes were mandatory, while participation in other sports or physical activities was highly encouraged. The situation appears different today, however.

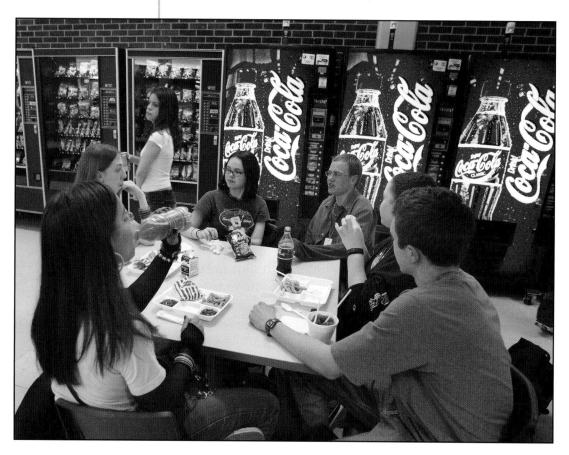

One example of the schools' relinquishing their opportunity to positively influence students' health habits occurred in 1989, when Channel One debuted. The brainchild of entrepreneur Chris Whittle, Channel One provided a daily 12-minute TV news broadcast to participating schools. Along with the news, however, came two minutes of ads, many of them for junk food and fast food. Educators soon realized that they had opened a Pandora's box of commercialism and junk food, similar to what children were watching on their own television sets at home.

Even so, Channel One has been adopted by 12,000 schools. Every school day, about 8 million children watch ads for products such as Pepsi, Hostess Twinkies, M&Ms, Snickers, and other junk-food products, which make up approximately 27 percent of Channel One's advertising. Channel One became a dream come true for junk-food marketers because of its captive audience sitting in a closed environment with no parents watching. Some school districts gave the marketers even further access to their students by allowing ads for various food products to be placed on school walls and in buses.

Once the guardians of good nutrition, some American schools now have become a haven for junk-food marketers in other ways as well. For instance, looking for a snack no longer means waiting until lunch or after school; it is only as far as the hallway vending machines. Nearly 19 out of 20 American high schools have vending machines that sell soda, while nearly 60 percent of elementary schools do. More than 70 percent of high schools sell chocolate candy in vending machines. Fast-food companies, too, now have a big presence in the schools, bypassing parents and promoting their high-fat products directly to children. At least one out of every five schools now contains a fast-food outlet.

In a Gallup Youth Survey poll taken in August 2003, teens were asked if they ever bought junk food or soda from school vending machines. Sixty-eight percent of those aged 13 to 17 reported that they had. Of that group, 71 percent of the boys bought vending-machine items, compared with 65 percent of the girls. In addition, 61 percent of the teens polled reported that they were more likely to eat some junk food every week; 23 percent reported that they ate a lot of junk food in the course of a week. Only 17 percent stated that they ate little or no junk food of any kind.

In the same survey, 13 percent of the teens polled said they were currently on a diet, with more girls (18 percent) than boys (9 percent) saying they were trying to lose weight. Many critics blame much of the teen eating problem on school vending machines. However, as some educators point out, restricting or eliminating vending machines from schools will not solve the problem completely; if junk food or fast food is not available at school, teenagers will simply look elsewhere to buy it. Teens agreed with this conclusion; in a 2004 Gallup Youth Survey poll, 68 percent of the teens responding believed that banning the sale of soda and junk food during school hours would prove largely ineffective in deterring students from buying junk food.

HARD TO TURN DOWN

In 1946 President Harry S. Truman signed the National School Lunch Act into law. Under its provisions, the government took on the responsibility of making sure students in American schools received at least one healthy and nutritious meal every day. As Truman stated, "The well nourished school child is a better student. He is healthier and more alert. He is developing good food habits that will benefit him for the rest of his life. In short, he is a better asset for his country in every way."

Today, more than 93,000 schools and 27.9 million children participate in the USDA-funded National School Lunch Program. Unfortunately, whereas administrators of school cafeterias once relied on in-house

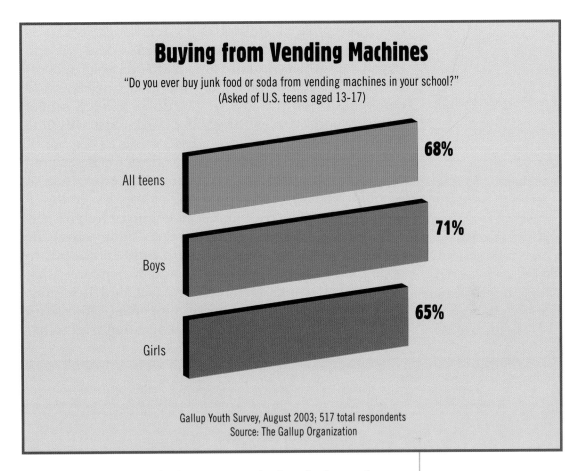

Buying from Vending Machines

"Do you ever buy junk food or soda from vending machines in your school?"
(Asked of U.S. teens aged 13-17)

All teens — 68%

Boys — 71%

Girls — 65%

Gallup Youth Survey, August 2003; 517 total respondents
Source: The Gallup Organization

cooks to prepare wholesome meals for their students, today cafeteria workers depend more on processed foods that they receive from the federal government. These foods in many ways are no better than what fast-food vendors offer. Also, while schools that receive federal support for their food-service operations are required to meet national nutrition guidelines, that does not mean vending machines or à la carte items sold in the cafeteria are restricted to healthy fare.

Even as angry parents, outraged newspaper editorialists, and exasperated health-care professionals complain about the presence of junk food in schools, the fact is that schools need the money they receive from these vendors. At stake, school officials maintain, are thousands of dollars from marketing contracts between schools and companies such as Coca-Cola and PepsiCo. With each bottle or can of soda sold, schools earn badly needed money to fund their programs and compensate for the loss of tax dollars. Even school organizations are getting on board; currently the National PTA lists Coca-Cola Enterprises as a sponsor.

When budget cuts hit a school, one of the first courses eliminated is physical education. The proportion of schools offering daily phys-ed classes in grades 9 through 12 declined from 42 percent in 1991 to 32 percent in 2001. Because funding is so tight across the nation, schools are often left with little choice but to open their doors to Channel One and to companies that promote soft drinks, junk food, and fast food. Ironically, with funds acquired from these companies, schools can put money back into physical education and other

An elementary school student in Massachusetts climbs high as part of a physical education and self-esteem program. When school budgets are tight, gym classes are often among the first programs to be cut.

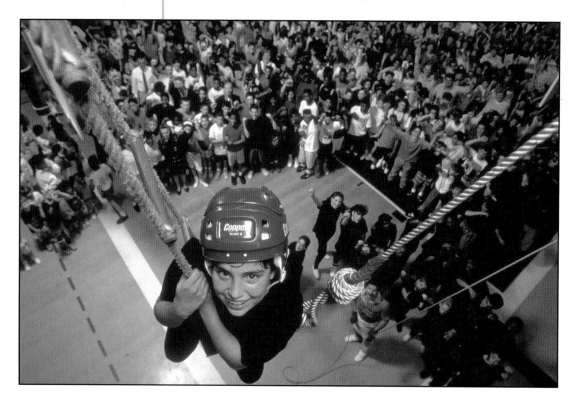

needed programs. It may be a devil's bargain, for the nation is waging an uphill fight against childhood obesity.

With only a few million dollars for ad campaigns to promote good nutrition, government agencies are overwhelmed by a fast-food industry that spends more than $3 billion a year on advertising, much of it directed toward children. In the last few years, however, many state legislatures have tried to limit the number of vending machines and fast-food outlets that can be placed in schools.

Winning the battle against childhood obesity — and preventing adult health problems related to excess weight before they strike — will take a concerted effort. Clearly, more programs are needed that provide education in good nutrition and that promote physical fitness. Such programs could go a long way in helping children learn how to live healthy lives.

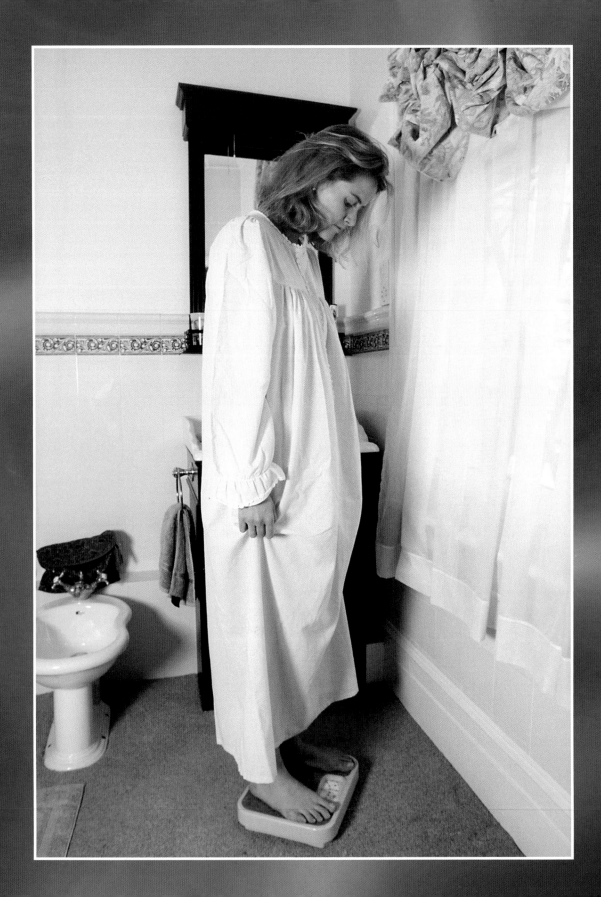

WHAT EPIDEMIC?

7

With the publication of the 2005 *JAMA* article disputing the government's figures on deaths attributable to excess weight, the debate over the obesity crisis reached another level. Experts hotly debated the data; many average Americans were confused about the nature and extent of the so-called obesity crisis. Did it really exist? Not for the first time, skeptics challenged the conventional wisdom of the federal government and the CDC.

FACT OR FICTION?

According to Paul Campos, author of *The Obesity Myth*, "There's this tremendous cultural hysteria about this issue which is really not justified at all by the scientific and medical literature." Campos and others contend that study after study has demonstrated that people who are overweight have a lower risk of premature death than those who are lean. Perhaps part of the reason is that fat provides additional energy in times of illness. Other studies have reported that people who intentionally lost huge amounts of weight died sooner than those who

(Opposite) Are Americans too obsessed with weight? Is the supposed "obesity epidemic" really just a myth? Some skeptics say yes.

stayed fat. The race to be thin may have a higher cost than previously thought, some believe.

Government agencies and obesity researchers objected strenuously to the analyses of Campos and like-minded critics. According to those who posit an obesity crisis, such critics are merely nitpicking over the data, ignoring studies that show unequivocally the harmful effects of obesity on a person's health.

THE B.M.I. FACTOR

Since the early 1950s, when the U.S. government began taking an expanded role in public health issues, some concerns were expressed about the small but growing number of overweight Americans. Yet even as the average weight of Americans continued to increase over the next three decades, no widespread alarm was raised. During the 1980s, as Americans ate out more often, relied more on prepared foods, watched more television, and spent longer hours in front of the computer, they gained weight more quickly than before. In 2004 the average American adult was 7 to 10 pounds heavier than the average American adult had been in 1990, with a typical man of five feet nine tipping the scales at 180 pounds, and a typical woman of five feet four weighing in at 154 pounds.

Skeptics do not dispute that Americans have gained weight; rather, they challenge the manner in which obesity is defined as well as its impact on health. Over the last 50 years, many health professionals have relied on weight tables and the body mass index (BMI) to gauge a person's "ideal" weight. Before 1998 a person with a BMI of 27 or above was considered overweight. As additional research showed the health risks posed by being overweight, the National Institutes of Health lowered the cutoff point to 25, the figure that the World Health Organization (WHO) already had adopted. At the same time, the cutoff point for obesity became a BMI of 30.

Overnight, about 30 million Americans were now classified as overweight—without having gained a pound. With the new guidelines in place, even a professional athlete like basketball star Shaquille O'Neal fell into the "obese" category because his muscle mass made his BMI number larger. To skeptics, this demonstrated that the BMI test, while helpful, should not be the central tool in discerning whether a person is overweight, obese, or normal.

THE DOUBTERS' CASE

Jeffrey Friedman, a molecular geneticist at the Rockefeller University, also believes that the "obesity

Pervasive images of slender models, actresses, and other glamorous figures may cause adolescent girls, in particular, to internalize the message that thin is beautiful. Unrealistic body images, in turn, can lead to eating disorders.

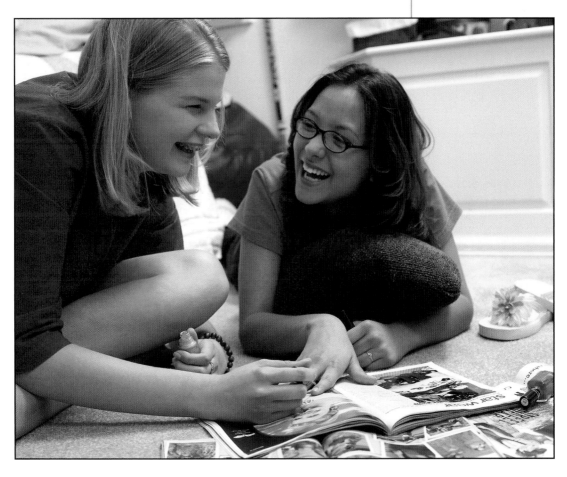

crisis" is more illusory than real, but for a different reason. Friedman concedes that the average weight of Americans has risen in recent decades, but he believes the statistical picture has been skewed by very large weight gains among a limited number of people: the very obese. The majority of Americans, he thinks, have remained about the same size, at most putting on a few pounds. Thus in Friedman's view it doesn't make sense to speak of an obesity epidemic or an obesity crisis, as the problem only affects a small minority (who happen to be genetically predisposed to excessive weight gain, a predisposition that is likely to play out in a society where food is abundant and sedentary lifestyles prevail).

Many critics see the issue of obesity in political, rather than simply medical, terms. They contend not only that the notion of an obesity epidemic is rooted in flawed data, but also that it is sustained by activists pushing an agenda of expanded government. These activists, critics charge, want legislation and other measures to punish the food industry and even impose taxes on consumers who make the "wrong" food choices. Needless to say, this charge inflames passions, as many Americans don't think government has any right to tell them what they should or shouldn't eat.

Barry Glassner, a sociology professor at the University of Southern California, has noted that the anxiety over the so-called obesity epidemic is similar to the media frenzy over flesh-eating bacteria, killer bees, and other health scares. Further, Glassner states, "from the hysteria from government officials and the media, one could easily get the impression that gaining a few pounds is the equivalent of taking up smoking or removing the seat belts from your car."

Campos also points out that the crusade against obesity is not just about keeping people thin, fit, and healthy; it also allows activists in the cause to express their aesthetic distaste for fat people. As Campos explained to *Los Angeles Times* reporter Rosie Mestel, "People who would not have been considered fat in any other time and place are considered fat in this culture and are bombarded with all this nonsense about how they've got to do something about their pathological bodies."

Other researchers agree. Some have charged that data collected by the CDC and other groups has been tainted by the prejudice against the obese. Further, skeptics point to a number of studies that provide evidence that overweight and obese people live longer than those who are thin. One example is a 2000 study of nearly 8,000 Europeans. Based on the data, thin men (with a BMI of less than 18.5) had twice the rate of death as overweight men.

Skeptics also complain that dieting is unhealthy. For instance, some population studies have reported that people who deliberately lost weight lived no longer than if they had stayed fat. Other studies have shown that people who lost weight died sooner. Still, while the CDC has backed away from previous estimates blaming obesity for up to 400,000 deaths in the United States annually, it still insists that an obesity epidemic exists: more than 100,000 Americans, the CDC said in 2005, die prematurely each year because they are very overweight.

BIG IS BEAUTIFUL

While the debate rages over whether an obesity epidemic exists in the United States, another solution has emerged for those who are overweight. Its emphasis remains on health and nutrition, but an important component has been added: self-acceptance. Today, there are organizations and groups dedicated to promoting self-esteem in overweight and obese people, as well as battling prejudice against those who are fat.

One of the first such groups to organize was the National Association to Advance Fat Acceptance

(NAAFA). Established in 1969, the group is a nonprofit human rights organization dedicated to improving the quality of life for fat people. NAAFA works to eliminate discrimination based on body size and provides fat people with education, advocacy, and member support. According to the group's website:

> We must also consider that in our society, it is very difficult for fat people to stay healthy and become fit. Due to prejudicial medical treatment and harassment by health care professionals, many fat people do not receive adequate preventative health care, and procrastinate seeking treatment when there is a medical problem. In addition, many fat people do not feel comfortable participating in activities that would lead to a greater level of fitness due to social stigma.

For NAAFA, then, the goal is to help fat people live normal lives in a society that often penalizes them for

The National Association to Advance Fat Acceptance sponsored this 1998 rally in Santa Monica, California, which the group lightheartedly dubbed the Million Pound March. Advocacy groups for the obese say fat people face routine discrimination in the United States.

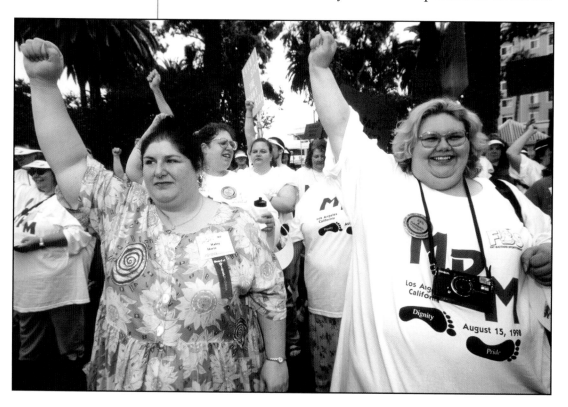

being overweight. When necessary, NAAFA has also gone to court to fight bias against fat people.

While NAAFA and other organizations provide help and support to obese persons of both sexes, women are a special focus. Given Americans' obsession with being thin, it was once difficult for larger-sized women to find products that took into account their weight. By the 1980s much of that had changed as marketing directors for clothing stores and other retail outlets realized there was an untapped market of potential customers. Today, a host of products and services are available for heavy women, including clothing lines, beauty products, magazines, and websites.

Meanwhile, as the two factions continue to argue over whether an obesity epidemic exists, Americans still struggle to make sense of the contradictory information with which they have been inundated. Most Americans are looking for balanced information, especially when it comes to nutrition and diet. With all the information available, however, many Americans often feel overwhelmed. In a Gallup poll conducted in 2002, about one in four (24 percent) of those surveyed reported difficulty in keeping up with information about eating a healthy diet. The fact is that many Americans simply want information about how to eat better.

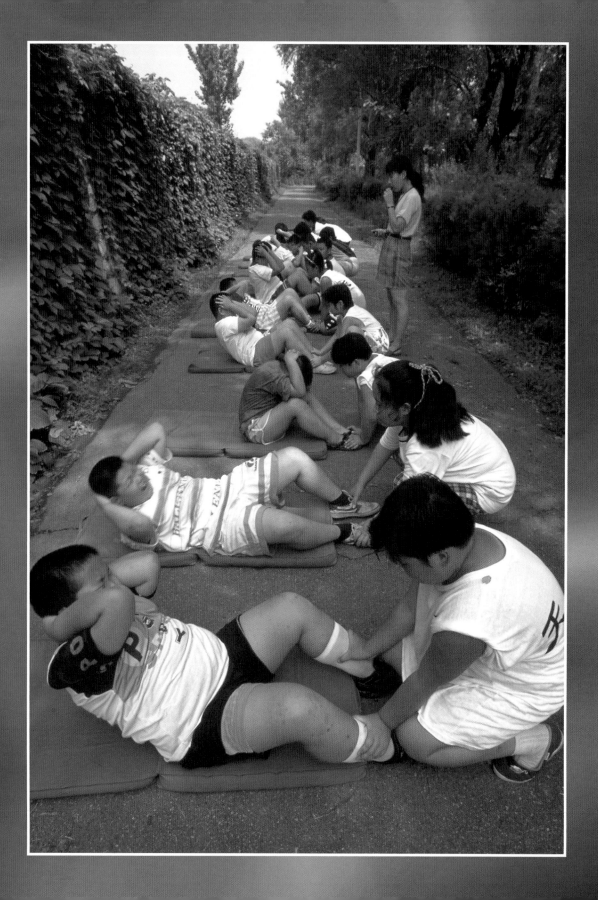

8

WE ARE THE WORLD: THE GLOBAL IMPACT OF OBESITY

In 2000 the World Health Organization declared obesity an "epidemic." In 2004, according to International Obesity Task Force statistics, approximately 1.3 billion persons in the world were overweight. Of those, about 312 million were classified as obese.

Although Americans are the heaviest, people in other Western countries have shown an increased tendency to be overweight. In Asia, Latin America, and elsewhere in the developing world, the number of overweight and obese people is also increasing. And in some countries of Africa and Southeast Asia, as well as parts of India, there is the spectacle of growing rates of obesity alongside widespread malnutrition.

IS AMERICA TO BLAME?

On the surface, it seems only natural to blame the United States for the increase in global obesity. After all, the eating habits of Europeans and

Chinese youngsters do sit-ups at a weight loss camp near Beijing. Obesity is increasingly becoming a global problem, even in societies in which a significant portion of the population suffers from chronic malnutrition.

Asians have changed largely as a result of the introduction of processed foods, fast-food franchises such as McDonald's and Burger King, and high-sugar products such as Coke, Pepsi, and candy.

In recent decades, U.S. food companies have increased their presence overseas. In Great Britain, the number of fast-food outlets doubled between 1984 and 1993; in France, a new McDonald's opens every five days. In Italy, tourists and natives easily can bypass the traditional Mediterranean diet of fish, fruit, and vegetables for less healthful fare from a Dunkin' Donuts or a McDonald's. Once the first Burger King opened in Milan, plans were made for a hundred more to open within three years. Throughout Europe, "American-size" portions and all-you-can-eat buffets are becoming popular, as are packaged and prepared foods. "There were good eating habits in this country at one time," says Professor Michele Carruba, director of the Research Center on Obesity at the University of Milan, "but unfortunately we're losing them pretty quickly."

Still, while many people point to America's role in global obesity, there is plenty of blame to go around. "America has been a contributing cause in what is a very complex disease," says Jim Mann, an expert on global obesity and a nutrition professor at the University of Otago in New Zealand. "But [America] is not the cause. Nothing is as simple as that." Even as Western consumerism and materialism have permeated cultures and societies around the world, experts point out that, for the most part, other nations and peoples have welcomed these changes. In fact, American food has replaced cigarettes as the cool, must-have American accessory.

The global impact of Western food is not a new area of study; more than 70 years ago, Dr. Weston Price, a dentist, traveled around the world studying diverse cultures. His findings stunned the medical establishment. Specifically, Price discovered that in multigenerational families where two mainstays of the Western diet—sugar and refined flour—were introduced, the health of the children underwent dramatic changes. For instance, facial and jaw structures narrowed, and the children were more prone to illness. Clearly, ingesting processed foods had a significant impact on how people looked and felt.

With so many American foods available globally and consisting of sugar, fat, refined carbohydrates, and animal protein, problems were likely to occur. As more people have chosen to eat like Americans, they also have had to deal with health problems that are similar to Americans'. Too little physical activity combined with cheap, high-calorie, high-fat foods is clearly taking a toll on the peoples of the world. As more than one

Company executives at the opening of the first Burger King franchise in Brazil, São Paolo, November 2004. In addition to its TV shows, movies, and music, the United States has succeeded in exporting its eating habits to much of the world.

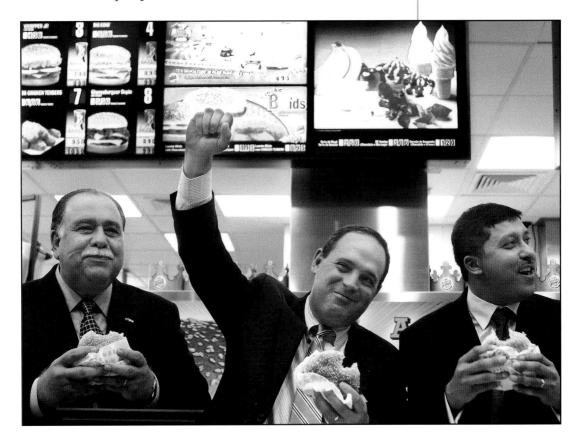

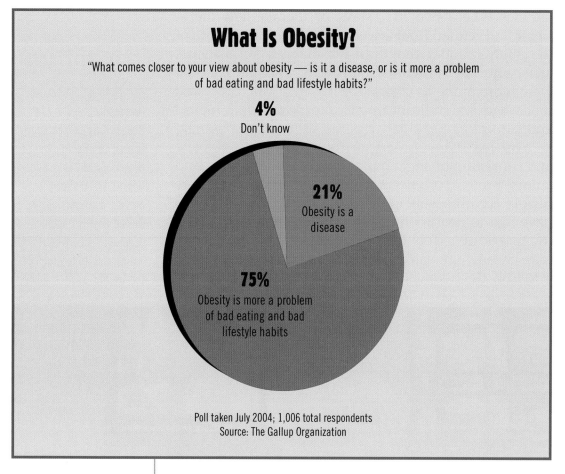

What Is Obesity?

"What comes closer to your view about obesity — is it a disease, or is it more a problem of bad eating and bad lifestyle habits?"

4%
Don't know

21%
Obesity is a disease

75%
Obesity is more a problem of bad eating and bad lifestyle habits

Poll taken July 2004; 1,006 total respondents
Source: The Gallup Organization

authority has pointed out, people still have the ability to make individual choices about what they eat. If they choose to eat fast food, prepared foods, or junk food on a regular basis, that is their decision. But such a viewpoint fails to confront the problem. Foreign governments need to address the fact that healthy food choices are both expensive and sometimes hard to find; as for physical activity, not all countries can make available resources such as those found in the United States.

POSSIBLE SOLUTIONS

In May 2004 the World Health Organization met with representatives of many nations and food companies to discuss the obesity epidemic. The WHO unveiled a strategy in which governments would work to discourage food and beverage ads that exploit the vulnerability of children; tax less-healthy foods more heavily; limit high-fat, high-sugar foods in schools; and review agricultural policies that may contribute to obesity, heart disease, diabetes, and cancer. The recommendations also suggested that people limit the amount of fat, sugar, and salt in their diets while increasing their consumption of fruits, vegetables, whole grains, beans, and nuts. Finally, the WHO urged all men, women, and children to engage in at least 30 minutes of moderate exercise almost every day.

Although the plan is not binding, the WHO hopes that governments will take the recommendations seriously and implement their own solutions to combat obesity. But experts believe that the WHO has no intention of stopping there; they expect the organization to begin pressuring food companies and advertising firms in the United States and around the world to promote good nutrition and healthy eating habits.

In some quarters there is concern that certain governments, bowing to the powerful food and restaurant industries in their countries, will attempt to soften the WHO recommendations. In 2005, for example, U.S. president George W. Bush was continuing to suggest changes to the WHO proposal, emphasizing greater personal, and less corporate, responsibility and limiting government intervention. As a member of the Washington-based Center for Science in the Public Interest noted, "No one is suggesting that government regulate what foods people put in their mouths, but the WHO recognizes that government has a role in making the healthy choice the easy choice."

Schools, too, have a role in promoting healthy lifestyles, and many are beginning to reexamine their policies. Some schools have removed junk food and soft drinks from vending machines and instead are stocking healthier snacks, fruit, juices, and water. Others have partnered with health-food companies to prepare healthy meals for student lunches. Finally, schools are investigating ways to raise money without relying on revenue generated from vending-machine contracts.

Responding to the calls of health-conscious consumers, fast-food companies have also begun changing their menus, adding salads and fruit. Children's meals at these restaurants have taken a turn for the better, with milk, juice, and fruit supplementing the requisite burger. McDonald's announced in 2004 that it no longer would offer customers the option of supersizing meals, and other restaurants are following suit. Additionally, food companies have taken steps to make snacks healthier by removing trans fats, one of the more harmful forms of fat that people ingest. New and improved

Fast-food companies have recently responded to calls for more healthful menu items. Here teens at a Wendy's in Illinois sample the restaurant chain's new fruit cups, February 2005.

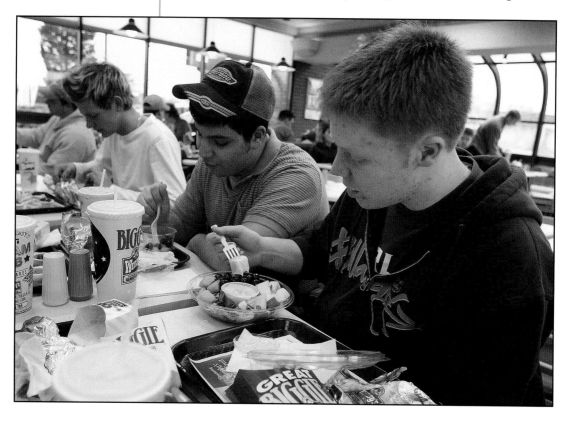

sugar substitutes such as Splenda, which are similar in taste and texture to real sugar, present viable alternatives as well.

Despite the positive roles that can be played by government, schools, and food companies, however, the battle against obesity must ultimately be waged by individuals. Those who make an effort to eat sensibly and exercise can greatly increase their chances of enjoying a healthier life. At the same time, acceptance of one's appearance, the gradual breaking down of stereotypes that stigmatize obesity, and the abandonment of unrealistic and unhealthy ideals of thinness can help Americans deal with weight issues in a more sensible and mature way. When Paul Campos was asked what Americans should do about obesity, he said they should stop obsessing about it. In other words, by being realistic and eating prudently, Americans can look forward to a healthier future, one meal at a time.

balanced diet—a combination of foods that, when consumed in appropriate amounts, provide all the essential nutrients to support growth and good health without weight gain.

body mass index (BMI)—a mathematical formula (BMI = kg/m^2) based on height and weight that is used to gauge whether someone is of normal weight, overweight, or obese.

calorie—a unit of heat that is used to measure the amount of energy a food can yield as it passes through the body.

carbohydrates—compounds that are produced mainly by plants and that constitute the major dietary source of energy; carbohydrates include sugars and starches.

cholesterol—a fat-like substance made by the body that is also found in food products from animals, such as meat, fish, poultry, eggs, and dairy products, and that can clog arteries.

diabetes—a disease in which the body's production and use of insulin (the hormone that enables the body to use and regulate sugar for energy) is impaired, causing sugar to build up in the bloodstream.

fast food—food, such as hamburgers, french fries, pizza, and fried chicken, that is prepared and served quickly by restaurants, typically for a relatively inexpensive price.

gastric bypass—a surgical procedure, performed in order to promote weight loss, in which most of the stomach is stapled closed, leaving a tiny remnant of stomach connected to the upper intestine.

genetic—caused or produced by hereditary as opposed to environmental factors.

gluttony—excess in eating or drinking.

heredity—the sum of characteristics genetically transmitted to an offspring from parents.

Medicaid—a U.S. government program providing health insurance to the poor.

Medicare—a U.S. government program providing health insurance to Americans age 65 or older.

morbid obesity—a condition in which being overweight is likely to bring about major medical problems.

obesity—the condition of having significantly more body fat as a percentage of body weight than is normal.

saturated fat—a fat found in animal and dairy foods that, if consumed in large quantities, can cause weight gain, raise blood cholesterol, and increase the risk of heart disease.

sedentary—having low activity or exercise levels.

stigmatize—to identify or describe in terms that bring contempt or reproach.

trans fat—a type of fat (often found in fried, processed, and snack foods) that can cause weight gain, raise blood cholesterol, and increase the risk of heart disease.

Abramovitz, Melissa. *Obesity*. San Diego: Lucent Books, 2004.

Akers, Charlene. *Obesity*. San Diego: Greenhaven Press, 2000.

Gordon, Melanie Apel. *Let's Talk About Being Overweight*. San Diego: Greenhaven Press, 1998.

Ingram, Scott. *Want Fries with That? Obesity and the Supersizing of America*. New York: Franklin Watts, 2005.

Libal, Autumn. *Social Discrimination and Body Size: Too Big to Fit*. New York: Mason Crest Publishers, 2005.

Nakaya, Andrea C. *Obesity: Opposing Viewpoints*. San Diego: Greenhaven Press, 2005.

Spurlock, Morgan. *Don't Eat This Book: Fast Food and the Supersizing of America*. New York: Putnam Adult, 2005.

http://www.obesity.org

The website of the American Obesity Association provides information and resources about many obesity issues.

http://www.bodypositive.com

A site that focuses on positive body images, no matter what size.

http://www.cdc.gov/nccdphp/dnpa/obesity/trend/maps/index.htm

The CDC website provides current reports and statistics on obesity in the United States.

http://www.health.gov/dietaryguidelines/dga2000/document/frontcover.htm

A government site that explains the hows and whys of good nutrition.

http://www.cfsan.fda.gov/~dms/qa-nutq.html

Questions and answers about eating and nutrition and staying healthy.

http://www.nal.usda.gov/fnic/pubs/bibs/topics/weight/consumer.html

A list of resources, including articles, websites, and books dealing with weight loss and obesity.

http://hin.nhlbi.nih.gov/portion/

Explains healthy eating habits and the differences between a portion and a serving.

http://www.shapeup.org

How to stay in shape using a variety of different programs, activities, and exercises.

http://www.surgeongeneral.gov/topics/obesity/calltoaction/fact_glance.htm

Provides resources on nutrition and obesity.

http://www.gallup.com

The website of the national polling institute includes polling data and analyses on hundreds of topics.

BOOKS AND PERIODICALS

Barker, Paul. "America's Greatest Social Divide Is Not Between Rich and Poor, or Even Black and White." *New Statesman*, Sept. 6, 1996.

Brownell, Kelly D., and Katherine Battle Horgen. *Food Fight: The Inside Story of the Food Industry, America's Obesity Crisis and What We Can Do About It.* Chicago: Contemporary Books, 2004.

Critser, Greg. *Fat Land: How Americans Became the Fattest People in the World.* New York: Houghton Mifflin, 2003.

"Land of the Fat: It's Time to Shape Up: Europeans Are Facing an Obesity Crisis That May Only Get Worse." *Time International*, Oct. 25, 1999.

Lemonick, Michael D. "How We Grew So Big." *Time*, June 7, 2004.

Mestel, Rosie. "Worth Its Weight in Debate." *Los Angeles Times*, July 23, 2004.

Newman, Cathy. "Why Are We So Fat?" *National Geographic*, Aug. 2004.

Reilly, Rick. "The Fat of the Land." *Sports Illustrated*, Sept. 22, 2003.

Rimm, Sylvia, with Eric Rimm. *Rescuing the Emotional Lives of Our Overweight Children: What Our Kids Go Through—and How We Can Help.* Emmaus, Pa.: Rodale, 2004.

Squires, Sally. "Into Our Stomachs and Out of Our Minds." *Washington Post*, July 28, 2002.

Weber, Eugen. *A Modern History of Europe.* New York: W. W. Norton, 1971.

INTERNET SOURCES

"Dietguide: U.S. Contributes to Global Obesity, but Can't Take All the Blame." Phillyburbs.com, November 1, 2004. Located at: www.phillyburbs.com/pb-dyn/articlePrint.cfm?id=386220.

Dodge, Robert. "Obesity Issue Reaches into Politics, Pocketbooks." *Dallas Morning News* online, Nov. 7, 2003. Located at: www.tcjl.com/ArticlesStudies/article%20DMN%20obesity%2011-03.doc.

"From Wallet to Waistline: Supersized Portions May Be More Than You Bargained For, Says Report." Center for Science in the Public Interest, June 18, 2002. Located at: www.cspinet.org/new/200206181.html.

Hellmich, Nanci. "Health Agency Presents Global Plan to Fight Obesity." *USA Today*, March 17, 2005. Located at: www.usatoday.com/news/health/2004-05-17-who-obesity_x.htm.

Jabbour, Kamal. "Expanding American Waistline: Problem Has Two Faces." *Syracuse Post-Standard* online, Oct. 11, 1999. Located at: http://running.syr.edu/column/19991011.html.

Lambert, Craig. "The Way We Eat Now." *Harvard Magazine*, May–June 2004. Located at: www.harvard-magazine.com/on-line/050465.html.

"McDonald's Obesity Suit Thrown Out." CNN.com, Sept. 4, 2003. Located at: www.cnn.com/2003/LAW/09/04/mcdonalds.suit.

"Political Food Fight Over Fat." CBSNEWS.com, Aug. 25, 2003. Located at: http://cbsnews.com/stories/2003/08/25/health/main569957.shtml.

Robinson, Jennifer. "The Cost of Convenience." *UNLV Magazine*, Spring 2005. Located at: http://magazine.unlv.edu/Issues/Spring05/23cost.html.

Ruskin, Gary. "The Fast Food Trap: How Commercialism Creates Overweight Children." *Mothering*, Sept. 2003. Located at: www.mothering.com/articles/growing_child/food/fast_food.html.

Zacharias, Patricia. "Snap, Crackle and Profit—The Story Behind a Cereal Empire." *Detroit News* online. Located at: http://info.detnews.com/history/story/index.cfm?id=146&category=business.

AMERICAN DIETETIC ASSOCIATION

Consumer Education Team
216 West Jackson Boulevard
Chicago, IL 60606
(800) 877-1600, ext. 5000 (for publications)
(800) 366-1655 (for recorded food/nutrition messages)
Website: www.eatright.org/Public

The American Dietetic Association, the largest organization of nutrition professionals in the United States, promotes healthy eating.

COUNCIL ON SIZE & WEIGHT DISCRIMINATION, INC.

P.O. Box 305
Mt. Marion, NY 12456
(845) 679-1209
E-mail: info@cswd.org
Website: www.cswd.org

This not-for-profit organization describes its mission as "working to end discrimination against people who are heavier than average."

NATIONAL CENTER FOR CHRONIC DISEASE PREVENTION AND HEALTH PROMOTION

Nutrition and Physical Activity
1600 Clifton Rd.
Atlanta, GA 30333
(404) 639-3534 or (800) 311-3435
Website: www.cdc.gov/nccdphp/dnpa

Under the auspices of the Centers for Disease Control and Prevention (CDC), the National Center for Chronic Disease Prevention and Health Promotion fosters better nutrition and exercise habits.

NATIONAL INSTITUTES OF HEALTH

U.S. Department of Health and Human Services
200 Independence Ave., SW
Washington, DC 20201

(877) 696-6775
Website: http://health.nih.gov/result.asp/476

The NIH offers information on a wide range of topics related to obesity and health.

NORTH AMERICAN ASSOCIATION FOR THE STUDY OF OBESITY

8630 Fenton St.
Silver Spring, MD 20910
(301) 563-6526
Website: www.naaso.org

Founded in 1982, this scientific society encourages research on the causes and treatment of obesity.

UNITED STATES DEPARTMENT OF AGRICULTURE

Food and Nutrition Center
1400 Independence Ave., SW
Washington, DC 20250
Website: www.usda.gov/wps/portal/usdahome

Among its many tasks, the USDA provides information and advice on proper nutrition, including the food pyramid.

WEIGHT-CONTROL INFORMATION NETWORK

1 WIN Way
Bethesda, MD 20892-3665
(877) 946-4627
E-mail: win@info.niddk.nih.gov
Website: http://win.niddk.nih.gov/index.htm

WIN, a service of the National Institute of Diabetes and Digestive and Kidney Diseases (NIDDK), provides up-to-date and scientifically sound information to the general public, health professionals, the media, and Congress on weight control, obesity, physical activity, and related nutritional issues.

Numbers in ***bold italics*** refer to captions.

Page:
3:      William Thomas Cain/Getty Images
8:      Tim Boyle/Getty Images
12:     Centers for Disease Control and Prevention, U.S. Department of Health
            and Human Services
15:     © OTTN Publishing
18:     Mark Wilson/Getty Images
20:     Library of Congress
24:     Time Life Pictures/Mansell/Time Life Pictures/Getty Images
27:     Fox Photos/Getty Images
29:     © OTTN Publishing
30:     Tim Boyle/Getty Images
32-33: Jana Birchum/Getty Images
36:     © OTTN Publishing
37:     © OTTN Publishing
39:     PhotoDisc
40:     Michelle Lawlor
42:     Spencer Platt/Getty Images
46:     U.S. Department of Agriculture
49:     William Thomas Cain/Getty Images
52:     Dolan Halbrook
54:     © OTTN Publishing
56:     Tim Boyle/Getty Images
61:     Roberto Brosan/Time Life Pictures/Getty Images
64:     James Keyser/Time Life Pictures/Getty Images
66:     Tim Boyle/Getty Images
68:     PhotoDisc
70:     Peter Parks/AFP/Getty Images
73:     Mike Fuentes/Getty Images
76:     Tim Boyle/Getty Images
79:     © OTTN Publishing
80:     Steve Liss/Time Life Pictures/Getty Images
82:     PhotoDisc
85:     Corbis Images
88:     Gilles Mingasson/Liaison/Getty Images
90:     Forrest Anderson/Time Life Pictures/Getty Images
93:     Mauricio Lima/AFP/Getty Images
94:     © OTTN Publishing
96:     Tim Boyle/Getty Images

For almost three-quarters of a century, the GALLUP POLL has measured the attitudes and opinions of the American public about the major events and the most important political, social, and economic issues of the day. Founded in 1935 by Dr. George Gallup, the Gallup Poll was the world's first public opinion poll based on scientific sampling procedures. For most of its history, the Gallup Poll was sponsored by the nation's largest newspapers, which published two to four of Gallup's public opinion reports each week. Poll findings, which covered virtually every major news event and important issue facing the nation and the world, were reported in a variety of media. More recently, the poll has been conducted in partnership with CNN and USA Today. All of Gallup's findings, including many opinion trends dating back to the 1930s and 1940s, are accessible at www.gallup.com.

ALEC M. GALLUP is chairman of The Gallup Poll in the United States, and Chairman of The Gallup Organization Ltd. in Great Britain. He also serves as a director of The Gallup Organisation, Europe; Gallup China; and Gallup Hungary. He has been employed by Gallup since 1959 and has directed or played key roles in many of the company's most ambitious and innovative projects, including Gallup's 2002 "Survey of Nine Islamic Nations"; the "Global Cities Project"; the "Global Survey on Attitudes Towards AIDS"; the 25-nation "Health of The Planet Survey"; and the ongoing "Survey of Consumer Attitudes and Lifestyles in China." Mr. Gallup also oversees several annual "social audits," including "Black and White Relations in the United States," an investigation of attitudes and perceptions concerning the state of race relations, and "Survey of the Public's Attitudes Toward the Public Schools," which tracks attitudes on educational issues.

Mr. Gallup's educational background includes undergraduate work at Princeton University and the University of Iowa. He undertook graduate work in communications and journalism at Stanford University, and studied marketing and advertising research at New York University. His publications include *The Great American Success Story* (with George Gallup, Jr.; Dow Jones-Irwin, 1986), *Presidential Approval: A Source Book* (with George Edwards; Johns Hopkins University Press, 1990), and *The Gallup Poll Cumulative Index: Public Opinion* 1935–1997 (Scholarly Resources, 1999).

MEG GREENE is a writer and historian. She holds a B.S. in history from Lindenwood College, St. Charles, Missouri, and two master's degrees, an M.A. in history from the University of Nebraska at Omaha and an M.S. in historic preservation from the University of Vermont. She is the author of more than 30 books. Two of her books have won awards: *Slave Young, Slave Long: A History of American Slavery* was given a 1999 Honor Book Award for social studies books, grades seven to twelve, by the Society of School Librarians International. *Buttons, Bones, & the Organ Grinder's Monkey: Tales of Historical Archaeology* was named a Best Book for Teens by the New York Public Library in 2001. Ms. Greene makes her home in Virginia.